MARGARET H

Public Health
in
America

This is a volume in the Arno Press series

PUBLIC HEALTH
IN
AMERICA

Advisory Editor

Barbara Gutmann Rosenkrantz

Editorial Board

**Leona Baumgartner
James H. Cassedy
Arthur Jack Viseltear**

See last pages of this volume
for a complete list of titles.

ANIMALCULAR
AND
CRYPTOGAMIC THEORIES
ON THE
ORIGINS OF FEVERS

ARNO PRESS

A New York Times Company

New York / 1977

Editorial Supervision: JOSEPH CELLINI

Reprint Edition 1977 by Arno Press Inc.

Copyright © 1977 by Arno Press Inc.

On the Cryptogamous Origin of Malarious
  and Epidemic Fevers was reprinted from
  the University of Illinois Library.

PUBLIC HEALTH IN AMERICA
ISBN for complete set: 0-405-09804-9
See last pages of this volume for titles.

Manufactured in the United States of America

Publisher's Note: This book has been reprinted
from the best available copies.

Library of Congress Cataloging in Publication Data
Main entry under title:

Animalcular and cryptogamic theories on the origins of
    fevers.

    (Public health in America)
    Reprint of On the cryptogamous origin of malarious
and epidemic fevers, by J. K. Mitchell, first published
in 1849 by Lea and Blanchard, Philadelphia; of Memoir
on the nature of miasm and contagion, by J. L. Riddell,
first published in 1836 in the Western journal of medical
and physical science, Cincinnati; and of Yellow fever
contrasted with bilious fever, by J. C. Nott, first
published in 1848 in The New Orleans medical and
surgical journal. New Orleans.
    1. Fever--Etiology. I. Mitchell, John Kearsley,
1798-1858. On the cryptogamous origin of malarious and
epidemic fevers. 1977. II. Riddell, John Leonard,
1807-1867. Memoir on the nature of miasm and contagion.
1977. III. Nott, Josiah Clark, 1804-1873. Yellow
fever contrasted with bilious fever. 1977. IV. Series.
RC106.A54 1977   616'.047   76-40658
ISBN 0-405-09839-1

CONTENTS

ON THE

CRYPTOGAMOUS ORIGIN

OF

MALARIOUS AND EPIDEMIC

FEVERS.

BY

J. K. MITCHELL, A.M., M.D.,

PROFESSOR OF PRACTICAL MEDICINE IN THE JEFFERSON MEDICAL COLLEGE
OF PHILADELPHIA.

"It has also happened that reflecting men, guided by general ideas and analogies, have enunciated truths which, only at some future period, could command general acceptance and acknowledgment. This always has happened, and always will happen, when the direct proofs of such a truth are wanting."—BISCHOFF.
"The infection may be aptly compared to the *seeds of vegetables* or the eggs of animals, which require a nice concurrence of certain degrees of heat, moisture, rest, nutriment, &c., to animate them."—SIR GILBERT BLANE.

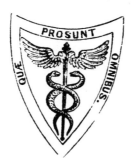

PHILADELPHIA:
LEA AND BLANCHARD.
1849.

PHILADELPHIA:
T. K. AND P. G. COLLINS, PRINTERS.

INTRODUCTION AND DEDICATION.

TO THE CANDIDATES FOR GRADUATION IN THE JEFFERSON
MEDICAL COLLEGE, OF THE SESSION OF 1846–1847:

GENTLEMEN:

To you, I had the honor of delivering, nearly in their present shape, the lectures which I now send to the press. Previously, I had not put my ideas on the subject of which they treat, into so formal a shape, although I had announced for years, to each successive class, my impression, that possibly, the protophytes might afford a good explanation of the causation of malarious, and other diseases of a febrile nature. Of the production thus, at least of yellow fever and cholera, I entertained less doubt, and taught, therefore, the sentiment with less reserve. But, although urged by some of you, and more formally requested by the class by which you were immediately succeeded, to place my opinions on this subject before the public, I refrained from their publication through aversion to controversy, and the hope that time would bring more conclusive evidence of their truth or falsehood. Other friends, whose age, position, and learning, entitled their opinions to the highest respect, did me the honor to listen to my elucidations, and to recommend their publication. Indeed, one of them, well known to you for his great learning and refined eloquence, wrote to Dr. Forbes, of

London, offering these lectures to him for his reprint of
American Medical Tracts. His plan, not embracing un-
published manuscripts, excluded them; but he kindly suggested the propriety of their immediate publication by
myself, as he thought an essay on a subject of so much
novelty ought not, through my aversion to publicity, to
remain inedited.

Since that time, a work of some merit has been printed
in England, and dedicated, by permission, to John Forbes,
M.D., by its author, Charles Cowdell, M.B., M.R.C.S.,
London, 1848. It professes to be, "*A Disquisition on
Pestilential Cholera,* being an attempt to explain its phenomena, nature, cause, prevention, and treatment, by reference to an extrinsic fungous origin." A review of
works on cholera, inclusive of that of Dr. Cowdell, appeared in the July number of the *British and Foreign
Medico-Chirurgical Review,* for 1848, in which the re-
viewer recommends to Dr. Cowdell to extend his hypothesis, which he thinks ingenious and interesting, "to
all epidemics. He would, perhaps, find yellow fever and
plague still more to his purpose than cholera."

Dr. Cowdell's book, and the review of it, reached me
nearly at the same time, and left me no further excuse for
withholding these lectures from the public, unless I pre-
ferred to lose what little of reputation might be obtained
by sending them to the press.

It will be seen that I have not attempted to conceal the
sentiments of former writers on this subject, although my
ignorance of German prevents me from knowing exactly,
how far the authors of that country, Henle, Müller, and
others, have carried their ideas. Nothing in Dr. Cowdell's book occurs to show that he was aware of any pre-
existent fungous theory of fevers, nor of the wide dissemi-

nation of that hypothesis on this side of the Atlantic; so that he is apparently entitled to the credit of having made, if not a new, at least an original theory of the cause of cholera.

As you have heard these lectures, gentlemen, you may not have forgotten that, in making my selection of facts and observations, I have, with a single exception, studiously avoided an appeal to phenomena perceived only by myself. I have created no facts for this subject; because I have long learned, as you will learn, to trust reservedly to alleged truths observed by a theorist, who cannot avoid, however just he may be, the coloring which, through a blinding partiality for a new discovery or hypothesis, is too often given.

I have not, however, been idle. Experiments are in progress which seem to promise more direct and unquestionable proof of the validity of our hypothesis; but they are yet incomplete, and therefore should not now appear, lest they might load so young a conception with a too dubious weight.

As there may, in the future, arise some dispute respecting the paternity of the theory which is now proposed, I may be indulged with the liberty of quoting the following extract from a letter by Professor J. W. Bailey, in answer to one from me:

" *West Point, March 5th*, 1845.

"Doctor J. K. Mitchell:

" My dear Sir: Please accept my thanks for your favor of the 29th ultimo. I was interested in your letter on the fungous origin of fevers; and it appears to me that you make out a very strong case, and one which appears more satisfactory than Liebig's somewhat vague ideas of 'communication of motion,' being the cause of the propagation of contagious poisons, fermentation, &c. Your theory will, at least, lead to experiment, while his, *if I comprehend it*, leads to nothing, and is only a way of saying that we don't understand the subject."

It would scarcely be proper, gentlemen, to overlook the kind note addressed to me by a committee from the class which immediately followed you, and which formed a principal inducement for correcting for the press, the following lectures.

"*Jefferson Medical College, December 8th*, 1847.

"PROFESSOR MITCHELL.

"Sir: At a meeting of the class held last evening, the following resolution was unanimously adopted:

"'Resolved—That a committee be appointed to wait upon Professor Mitchell, and request him to furnish for publication, his new and original views of the nature and cause of malarious diseases.'

"Allow us, in fulfilling the agreeable duty imposed by the class, to express the high gratification we have derived from listening to the lectures referred to, and to add our personal solicitations that you will grant the favor which it is the object of the resolution to ask.

"Yours respectfully,

"W. P. THORNTON, of Mississippi.

"R. S. HAYNES, of Virginia.

"JNO. HORACE SELTZER, of Pennsylvania.

"CHAS. F. STANSBURY, of the District of Columbia, Chairman.

"JOHN O. McREYNOLDS, of Kentucky, Secretary."

In reply to this kind request, I promised, when at leisure, to cause the lectures to be published; and now commence the work by offering to you, who heard them first, in the form and substance in which they now appear, a dedication of them. With the most sincere desire for the promotion of your welfare, and with the greatest respect,

I have the honor to be, Gentlemen,

Your friend and preceptor,

J. K. MITCHELL.

TABLE OF CONTENTS.

ON THE

CRYPTOGAMOUS ORIGIN

OF

MALARIOUS AND EPIDEMIC FEVERS.

~~~~~~~~~~~~~

LECTURE I.

THEORIES OF MALARIA.

THE most ancient authors allude to the noxious influence of the air of marshes and stagnant pools. Some of them indulge in speculations respecting the immediate cause of its morbific power; and here and there, in their writings, may be detected, more or less vaguely expressed by them, the opinions, by the publication of which, Lancisi, less than two centuries ago, acquired so much reputation. His treatise *de noxiis paludum effluviis*, gave consistency and authority to the impression of the miasmatists, and the loose idea of a former age, became the accepted sentiment of the eighteenth century. By degrees, the medical profession, almost everywhere, adopted the theory of the causation of periodical fevers by marsh air, and even ascribed the poison to a decomposition of the vegetable remains of low and wet places. After that time (1695),

2

with occasional modification from the fancy of each author, the vegetable theory of miasm became almost an established dogma of the schools, not often questioned until the very time in which we live. Now, writers, dissatisfied with the inexact condition of the subject, demand proofs in favor of the marsh theory, which they cannot find; and I may, perhaps, feel safe in asserting, that, at the present day, few well-informed physicians accept the theory of the miasmatists, as detailed by McCulloch.

Whatever view may be taken of the nature of the pestilential cause, it is usually most potent in places of a moist and marshy character, such as are the borders of lakes and rivers; and in such places it commonly most abounds, when accompanied by a luxuriant vegetation and a high temperature. As heat, moisture, and vegetation, so commonly attend the production of malarious influence, careless observers, naturally enough, believe the action of heat and moisture upon the vegetation, to be the efficient cause of miasm; while they refer to contrasts of temperature and moisture as exhibited by day and night, as the exciting causes of the periodical fevers of such places.

Such conditions, predisposing and exciting, no doubt cause such maladies; but inquirers take very different views of the mode of production, and of the immediate agents concerned. Some conceive, as already stated, that by decomposition, a predisposing poison is produced, sufficient of itself often to excite disease, whilst dews and change of temperature may occasionally precipitate or determine an attack. Others think that the mephitic vapors of marshes only enfeeble health, and thus enable the obvious changes of heat and moisture to excite disease, which they often produce without any such preparation.

A third party refers all cases of periodical disease exclusively to sensible changes, and thinks the proximity of a marsh only efficient as presenting an evaporating surface, by which the air is made colder and damper.

Dissatisfied for many reasons, to be hereafter offered, with the vegetable theory, and with the evaporating theory, and indeed with the hypothesis by which both are united, authors of our own time have suggested a variety of explanations, which it may not be inexpedient to pass in cursory review.

The commonly received marsh theory is well stated and supported by McCulloch, to whose work on malaria I refer you for a view of that side of the question. It is, in a much more masterly and precise manner, sustained by Dr. Craigie, of Edinburgh, to whose volumes on the Practice of Medicine, you may most profitably resort for a learned, lucid and, I think, impartial array of the facts and opinions bearing on that side of the question. McCulloch involves himself in difficulties without seeming to see them, whilst Craigie, although inclined to the same conclusions, views with a master's eye, the whole of the impediments and objections. The objections presented by the latter are: the low temperature at which these disease-producing changes may take place; the unaccountable production of them in places where there is no apparent vegetation and often no marsh; the exemption of certain places where occur all the seeming elements of decomposition; the inexplicable effects of rural cultivation; and the unexplained vicissitudes of health in the same places in different though similar years.

Denying the vegetable theory, and indeed assuming the position that we are as yet totally ignorant of the nature and true source of the cause of malarious fevers, my eminent colleague, Professor Dunglison, in his work on Hygiene, ably exposes the fallacy of the received opinions on this subject. He is not favorably impressed, indeed, by *any* of the many hypotheses with which an obscure, but highly important subject like this, is sure to be loaded.

Not less antagonistic to the received theory, is my friend, Dr. John Bell, who, however ingenious and learned in his opposition to it, does not also arrive at a negative conclusion, but refers the morbid phenomena to the modification of the sensible or appreciable conditions of the atmosphere. His paper, contained in the *Medical and Physical Journal*, for 1825, 1826, pp. 274–316, is worthy of an attentive perusal, although written at a very early period of his medical life.

Notwithstanding, therefore, the seeming supererogation, my duty as a teacher compels me to offer to you at least a summary of the objections to current opinions on this subject.

The most forcible argument against the vegeto-aerial theory, consists in the extraordinary exemption from malarious diseases of places which, were it true, could not escape a severe infliction. It is the more forcible, because the theory is founded mainly upon the concurrence of such diseases with heat, moisture and vegetation. If, then, it can be shown that the alleged conditions exist in the most perfect state, *in very many places*, without morbid results, the universality of the coincidence can no longer be brought to sustain the opinion.

Again, if *many places* can be cited, where these supposed elements are not at work, which are nevertheless noted for their insalubrity, the opinion becomes even less tenable. It is still farther weakened by the fact, often observed, that under precisely the same apparent circumstances, healthy places become unhealthy, and sickly places, salubrious. The marsh, the heat, the moisture and the vegetation, remaining apparently the same, the health of a region may vary from one extreme to the other.

I will now offer you some examples in illustration of these positions:

McCulloch, the unqualified advocate of the Marsh theory, seems to have been very much perplexed by an exception to his rule, which lay just under his own eye. The canal in St. James' Park, London, was, at the time he wrote, notorious for the abundance of its aquatic plants, causing, in autumn, an even intolerable stench. Yet he congratulates the inhabitants, on their miraculous exemption from malarious fevers, "it being, perhaps, *the only exception in the world,* at least wherever the climate equals (in temperature) that of England."—(p. 50.)

Let us see how far his assertion is sustainable. The town of Kingston, in the island of St. Vincent, is situated at the bottom of a semicircular bay, and at the foot of a mountain range, with high land on each side. The soil consists of a black alluvial mould, evidently arising from decaying vegetable matter. In one place, the bed of a dried up water-course, branches of trees were found, and the neighboring ground was covered with leaves, in different stages of decomposition, for upwards of eight inches in depth, into which the feet sank at every step. "There, then," says the deputy inspector of British hospitals and fleets, Robert Armstrong, "we have all the elements necessary for the production of this vegeto-animal poison, heat, moisture, decayed and decaying vegetable matter, with as large a proportion of reptiles, insects and other animal matters, as is found in other tropical countries; yet strange to say, the town of Kingston is one of the most

2*

healthy spots in the West Indies. I was informed by the staff-surgeon to the forces, who had long resided there, that *it was as healthy as the most favored spots in England*." As a very curious contrast to the statement of Armstrong, we learn from Bishop Heber, that the wood tracts of Nepaul and Malwa, *having neither swamps nor perceptible moisture*, become in summer and autumn, so pestiferous as to cause their abandonment even by the birds and beasts.

Fordyce too, tells us that, in a part of Peru, where there is almost a total absence of water, and of course of vegetation, fever and dysenteries render the country almost uninhabitable; and according to Pringle, the dry unproductive sandy plains of Brabant, excite malarious fevers of great intensity.

New South Wales extends from 10° 5' to 38° south latitude, embracing a region similarly situated to that of America from the West Indies to the Chesapeake Bay. It is subject to a rainy season, has streams, estuaries, and extensive swamps. Around some of its towns there lies a deep, black, highly productive vegetable mould. It is liable to extraordinary inundations, which lay the country, as far as the eye can reach, under a sheet of muddy water. The temperature is quite as high as that of any other like latitude. The coast is covered with *mangroves*, and skirted by rocks, reefs and islets. Among its products are mahogany, oranges, lemons, guavas. The mosquito, with myriads of insects and reptiles; parrots, paroquets and other tropical birds, announce a hot, productive climate, and lead us to look for a tainted air and a pestilential habitude. But, notwithstanding all these threatening conditions, the usual symbols of a sickly clime, New Holland is remarkable for its healthfulness. Pulmonary diseases and, in the wet season, dysenteries are observed, but the fevers incident to warm climates elsewhere, are here of rare occurrence. In speaking of this country, Malte Brun has this expression: " Hitherto we have heard of no such fatal epidemic fevers as are frequent in some other colonies situated in warm climates."

Mr. Titian Peale, the zealous and successful naturalist, who accompanied Captain Wilkes on the exploring expedition to the Southern Ocean, writes to Professor Dunglison, that he *never* saw a case of intermitting fever in either natives or strangers, in the Polynesian Islands, although the officers and men of the expedition lived and slept in the midst of marsh stenches and mosquitoes, when the days were hot, and the huts open and exposed.

Captain Wilkes himself describes these islands as fertile, moist, hot,—but, yet as remarkably salubrious, as is evinced by the general good health of the men, who were often exposed at night, by the shore duties of the service, to fatigue, night air and heavy dews.

The following examples of the truth of his general statement, are found in the same work.

TONGATABOO is an *organic island*, formed by coral, is *rich, flat* and *luxuriant*, and oppressed by a temperature rising to 98° F., offering a mean, during the sojourn of the expedition, of 79° 25. There was much rain, and, when clear, heavy dews. The writer supposes that these phenomena must create sickness, but he sees *many old* people, and admits that, *although ashore at night*, the people of the expedition were not sufferers. Mr. Peale, also, testifies to the good health of the place.

OVOLAU (Fegee) is a *volcanic island*, the mean temperature of which, for six weeks, was 77° 81; maximum, 96°; minimum, 62°. Turnips, radishes, and mustard seed appeared above ground in twenty-four hours; melons in three days; while marrowfat peas, fit for use, were produced in five weeks. On this island, volcanic as Sardinia, and hot as the Maremma, "fevers, whether remittent or intermittent, were unknown."

In the two instances cited above, the islands closely resembled each other in climate, temperature, and fertility, but were contrasted as to origination, geology, and surface, the one being organic, the other volcanic; the one being flat, the other mountainous; yet both enjoyed a degree of salubrity totally at variance with our preconceptions.

The Island of Soloo, in latitude 6° 01' North, enjoys a temperature seldom below 70°, or above 90°; that is, about the mean of that of the pestilential western coast of Africa. It is, however, healthy.

Menouf, the capital of Menoufyez, in Lower Egypt, is situated on the banks of a canal formerly navigable, but so no longer. This canal bathes the walls of Menouf from south to west. Within a few yards of it lies another canal of stagnant water, the space between, forming a road into the town. To the right of the south gate, lie basins of water *to rot flax in*, which gave out a disagreeable odor. Here and there is a cemetery, and between them are pools for the same use, some of them broken, neglected, and full of stagnant water. Menouf has no gardens, its streets are narrow and dirty, and its houses small and badly constructed. The people drink the Nile water. The yearly inundation floods the country around Menouf, up to the walls, but it does not continue long under water, to which fact Surgeon Carriè ascribes it healthfulness: " C'est pour cela sans doute que cette ville est assez saine."

In addition to its other defects, the place is surrounded

by a second wall, formed of dirt and rubbish, transported from town, by which the view is obstructed, and the town sheltered from the wind. Not only is Menouf *assez saine* in other respects, but even the plague does less damage here than in other parts of Egypt. (Degenettes.)

If the exception presented by the canal in St. James' Park puzzled McCulloch, and was, at the time he wrote that page, apparently, to him the only one, he alighted, in his progress, upon another, at Singapore, which seemed still harder to dispose of, without a severe shock to his system.

My esteemed friend and former pupil, Dr. M. B. Hope, Professor of Belles Lettres in the College at Princeton, resided for some time as a missionary at Singapore, in the East Indies, and adds to the details given by McCulloch, respecting Singapore, the following facts and opinions.

"The Island of Singapore is, in the main, *low* and *level*. There is one hill in the interior about 500 feet high, in which granite rocks make their appearance. Scattered here and there, are low round sand hills, the level ground between which is formed of a ferruginous clay upon a sandy substratum. The greater part of the island is covered with jungle. Lofty trees, and a most luxuriant vegetation are found in many places. The island is pretty well watered by streams, which descend from the hills to the sea. The tides have produced and sustained a chain of marshes nearly all round the coast. In some places, fresh and stagnant water covers the low grounds extensively.

"The city, which lies in latitude 1° 17', contains a highly mixed population of about 20,000 souls: Chinese, Malays, Indians, Europeans, &c. It is nearly surrounded by marshes, the jungles of which are almost impervious,

and are infested by tigers and other ferocious or wild
animals. Here and there the Chinese have cleared and
cultivated the ground; and there are, near the city, some
sugar and nutmeg plantations.

"The vegetation is incredibly rapid in its growth; and
its decay is not less wonderfully great, as may be supposed,
when the soil is rich, and the mean annual temperature
is, in the morning and evening, 79° 45', and at noon 84°.

"Astonishing as it may seem under such circumstances,
fevers *of any kind* were *very rare,* particularly among the
natives. Now and then remittent fevers might occur,
and, yet more rarely, intermittents. Foreigners were, of
course, more readily attacked, but not often, except
through imprudent exposure to fatigue, or the sun.

"Singapore is considered as a kind of *sanatarium* for
the Oriental invalids, who go thither from every quarter
of the Eastern world, to escape from malaria, or to recover from chronic diseases."

The empire of Brazil extends from the equator to the
southern tropic. It is watered by vast rivers and countless streams, abounds in lakes and marshes, and, under a
burning sun, smokes from the vapor of impetuous rains,
and boasts a vegetation unsurpassed for abundance, variety, and rapid transitions. Along an extended coast,
the mountain ranges are nearly parallel to the sea; so
that behind them the sea breeze exerts no cooling power,
and the air is stagnant and hot. Even at Rio Janeiro,
the latitude of which is nearly 23°, the temperature is
very high, and the atmosphere often excessively languid
and oppressive. "In the city," says Dr. Horner, of the
United States Naval Service (293), "the thermometer had
been 90 degrees in the shade. Night and day the temperature in my state-room was 86°." The sluggishness

of the air at Rio may be known by the name *Nitheroy*, or *Dead Sea*, given by the aborigines to its harbor. The climate is hot and moist; high and thickly wooded mountains, the narrow entrance to the bay, and the numerous islands impede the free passage of the wind." The site of the town is low, the streets are indescribably filthy, and the waters from the hills accumulate in the marshes which nearly encompass the city.—(*Hist. of Brazil.*) " The proximity of the ocean, the great size of the harbor, the great height of the land about it, the many hills, narrow streets, and high temperature, keep Rio, almost without cessation, immersed in a heavy, sultry atmosphere, rendered more disagreeable by want of cleanliness, and the exhalations from the ravines and marshy grounds in its rear." (Horner.)

Notwithstanding the presence of all the alleged *materiel* for fevers, the American squadron, with a mean force of 2,280 men, had, in 17 months, only 155 cases of fever, of which the Concord alone, had 70 in a crew of 200, when on a visit to the African coast. *Not one died of fever on the Brazil station.* The British ship Warspite, with a complement of 600 men, lay a whole year in the harbor of Rio, and did not lose a man. *In that time she had but seven cases of fever.*

Travelers who spent some time in Rio, and who penetrated to every part of the country, are equally warm in their praise of the salubrity of the climate. "It was," says Walsh, the rainy season, *a mortal period in other tropical climates.* For eight or nine hours a day, during some weeks, I never had dry clothes on me, and the clothes of which I divested myself at night, I put on quite wet in the morning. When it did not rain, there shone out in some places, a burning sun, and we went smoking along, the wet exhaling by heat, as if we were dissolving into vapor. Such weather in Africa, no human being could bear; but not so in Brazil; no one is affected by those states of the atmosphere which are so fatal elsewhere. It has, with some reason, therefore, grown into a proverb, that it is a country where a physician cannot live, and yet where he never dies. There was no doctor at S. Jose; but I was told there had been two at S. Joao d'el Rey, and that one of them had left because he could get no patients, and that the other had for a long time, no patient but himself."—(p. 297, vol. ii.)

In Africa, under the same latitude, the rains scarcely commence before the constitution begins to sink, even without external exposure. According to Lind, the first rains which fall in Guinea, are supposed to be the most unhealthy; *and they have been known in forty-eight hours, to render the leather of shoes quite mouldy and rotten.* Mungo Park observes, "that the rain had not commenced three minutes, before many of the soldiers were affected with vomiting, *others fell asleep, and seemed as if intoxicated.* I felt a strong inclination to sleep during the storm, and as soon as it was over, I fell asleep on the wet ground, although I used every exertion to keep myself awake. *Twelve of the soldiers were ill next day.*"

"The thermometer," says Boyle, "is seldom above 81°, or below 69° at this period, but the process of decomposition proceeds so rapidly, that cloth and animal substances, such as leather, become putrid in a period hardly credible."

On one of the Isles de Loss, at Sierra Leone, a small force was soon destroyed, yet it is in the sea, only about from half a mile to a mile in diameter, and formed *of granite,* which rises to three hundred feet at its centre.

It is apparently free from supposed causes of fever. There is but one piece of arable ground, no sulphur, no calcareous rock, no marsh, and very little soil, not a swamp, and the temperature seldom rises above 80°.—(Boyle, p. 16.)

Other examples almost without number, might be given of the salubrity of places full of decomposing matter, and of the insalubrity of others, where scarcely a vegetable is to be seen. So that many reflecting men are now disposed to abandon a theory, which cannot be rationally sustained by a reference to facts, and which is shaken the more, the more closely its pretensions are examined.

"We must be contented to place the explanation of the cause of plague," says Fodere, "in the category of that of all endemic maladies: that it is unknown."

"Malaria is a specific poison producing specific effects on the human body, and is probably gaseous or aeriform. Of its physical or chemical qualities, we really know nothing."—(Watson.)

According to Robert Armstrong, "we are utterly ignorant of the nature of this poison, and no two authors agree respecting its constitution, the circumstances under which it is generated, or its effects on the human body." —(p. 70.) Again, "of the existence of miasm we have no positive proof. It has never been obtained in an insulated state, and consequently, we are totally ignorant of its physical properties."

"If asked what is Malaria, I answer, I do not know." (Caldwell.)

"Hence, physicians have been reduced to the necessity of inferring the existence of hidden atmospheric influences, as a cloak for ignorance."—(Tweedie.)

"Epidemic fever may be attributed to a *mysterious*

3

something, an occult quality in the atmosphere."—(*Med. Gaz.*, xvi. p. 515.)

But thinking men can scarcely rest satisfied with negative conclusions, and therefore, new explanations of the cause of fever, succeed to the uprooted theories of the age gone by.

The opinion which, next to that of "the malarial," seems to be most successfully sustained, refers intermittents to the obvious conditions of the air, altered by heat and moisture; hot days followed by cool evenings, dry days, by dewy nights. The strongest argument for this conclusion, rests on the fact, that such diseases prevail at the season of greatest contrast, both as to heat and humidity, and in places where extensive wet grounds aid in the production of the strong vicissitudes.

As these phenomena are subject to observation, a close examination may be made of the relative condition in such respects, of the most healthy and the most deadly localities. The result is not favorable to the theory based on them, for many very salubrious places are remarkable for the most striking manifestations of the supposed causes of intermittents, while very sickly situations are not unfrequently distinguished by the uniformity of the climate, and the steadiness of the temperature and dew-point; nay, two places, in all observable respects alike in elevation, local relations, atmospheric phenomena and geological structure, may differ totally in their degree of healthfulness. Even in the same place, the line of limitation of disease-producing power, may be a common road, a narrow street, a stone wall, or a belt of woods; things which could scarcely be supposed to affect, sensibly, the heat and moisture, or their fluctuations.

But the most fatal argument against this theory is the

fact that exposure for a single hour, at night, sometimes produces an almost immediate attack in some persons, whilst in others it creates a tendency to disease, not actively expressed until the lapse sometimes of months. It will be acknowledged, too, that in that hour there may be observed no unusual or contrasted conditions of the air, either as to temperature or moisture.

On the western coast of Africa the sickness reaches its maximum in the height of the rainy season, when the diurnal temperature and moisture are almost invariable. Whilst on the coast of Brazil the same meteoric phenomena are perfectly innocuous.

Like every other theory, therefore, this one owes its plausibility rather to the defects of a former hypothesis than to its own value.

Daniel in England, and Gardiner in this country, have adopted, with slight modification, an opinion of Rammanzani, that marsh exhalations owe their injurious activity to sulphureous emanations. It is not enough to demonstrate their destructiveness, that their presence in minute quantity may be detected in paludal air; for the same argument would equally favor the reference of marsh fevers to any one of the many other gases or vapors found in the same places. The innocuous qualities of these as manifested elsewhere, is not less than those of the compounds containing sulphur. Moreover, the sulphureous localities of the sickly island of St. Lucia, are its only salubrious places.—(Evans.) Cities, too, which abound in sulphur-products, should not, according to this theory, enjoy the immunity from agues for which they are everywhere noted.

Immediately around the sulphur works and factories for making gunpowder and sulphuric acid, the vegetation and the ague disappear together. Facts of the same import might be almost indefinitely multiplied, but the task is unnecessary.

Hoffman attributed malarious fevers to a *lessened elasticity of the air*. His notion, obscurely conceived and inaccurately stated, is only excusable because of the loose philosophy of his day on every subject connected with atmospheric phenomena. Air is always equally elastic, and any modification of its density, except by adulteration, cannot be very partial for any length of time, so as to create a permanent insalubrity. When adulterated by excessive moisture or unusual gases, it is altered in composition, a cause of disease much more intelligible than that of modification merely of density.

Particular gases have also been supposed to exert malarious influence : Carbonic acid, nitrogen, cyanogen, carburetted hydrogen, phosphuretted hydrogen, ammonia and all the imaginable *effluvia* from decomposing organic compounds, have had, each, its advocate. As yet, however, no one has been able to show that marshy or insalubrious places abound most, or peculiarly, in such emanations; nor has it been made even probable that any one of these can, or ever did produce an ague ; while we know that in the busy haunts of non-malarial districts, the arts produce indefinitely diversified decompositions and emanations both animal and vegetable, with wonderful impunity to artisans.

The great difficulties in the way of other theories have induced some authors to suppose that the emanations productive of fevers result from the action on water of *living vegetables*, or of vegetables *not dead but dying*. Others have found more astringent vegetables in hot than in cold climates, and have conjectured that *some combination of animal matter with tannin constituted malaria*. Not yet satisfied with conjectures, a few presume that the decomposition merely of *certain* vegetables, forms or diversifies miasmata. " Thus," says McCulloch, "might *the cruciform plants*, OR THE TRIBE OF FUNGI, produce a malaria differing from that poison as resulting from the gramineous ones, or the consequence of the putrefaction of seeds differ from that of leaves." Some French writers lay great stress on the influence of *narcotic vegetables* in the causation of malaria.

McCulloch, after a very elaborate citation of facts and opinions, arrives at the *indefinite* conclusion "that the presence of *vegetables* or vegetable *matter*, in *some mode* or *form*, is necessary to the extrication of malaria; while the conclusion has sometimes been, that it is a production formed between *the living vegetable and water:* more generally that it is generated between *that* and the *latter*, *in some stage intermediate between life and absolute decomposition*; or, *lastly, that it is the consequence of absolute putrefaction*."

I need scarcely say that the ifs and ands, and buts and ors, in McCulloch's book, show the utter inefficiency of his undefined cause, to explain the difficulties of this vexed question. Nor is it necessary to offer objections to the other theories cited, since no one has sustained them by even plausible reasoning or pertinent facts. They are not received or respected by the 'profession.'

The last of the theories to which I shall invite your attention, are those of Drs. Ferguson and Robert Jackson.

The latter gentleman, once a firm believer in malaria as usually understood, saw, during his West India service, so many antagonistic phenomena as to incline him to the opinion, that it is, sometimes at least, *an emanation from living vegetables*, through the exuberance of organic life, the excess of vital vegetable action. To use his own language,

3*

"It would appear that the materials of vegetation abounding in excess, acted upon by a powerful cause, give out a principle, which, not being expended on the growth and nourishment of plants, is diffused to a certain extent in the atmosphere, causing a derangement of such bodies as come within the sphere of its action."

Mr. Doughty offers a modification of this sentiment, in the supposition that by the separation of their nutrition from the soil, especially when their growth is very rapid, plants cause in the earth new combinations of rejected elements, which thus become aerial, and poison the neighboring atmosphere. As many highly malarious places are barren, and naked of apparent vegetation, the theory of Jackson falls at once to the ground. But if not, then is there the additional difficulty of explaining by such a cause, the existence of malarious diseases when the season of active phenogamous vegetation has passed. It is also a pure hypothesis unsustained by facts or reasoning.

The theory of Ferguson is received now by the profession more favorably than perhaps any other. It narrows the malarial question down to this, that the only conditions essential to the production of miasmata are soil and water, especially a porous soil. And the only relation between these elements is, that of successive moisture and dryness. Stating it in the words of Dr. Watson, of London: "There is reason to believe that the flooding of a porous earthy surface with water, and a subsequent drying of that surface, under a certain degree of heat, constitute the sole or main conditions of the generation of the poison."

If these are the sole conditions, only moisture can come from the soil, for if anything else does, *it* must be a miasm, and we revert to the old opinion of Lancisi. If only moisture is exhaled, why does it sometimes poison its subjects in a single hour, or make an impression actively expressed sometimes months afterwards? Ferguson has himself adduced a fact irreconcilable with his theory, where the army suffered in long droughts when at a distance from porous and wet soils. His hypothesis is also in opposition to the fact that *in Africa the greatest mortality is during the rains,* when the earth is always drenched with water. On the other hand, the shores of the Mediterranean are most pestilential when a long drought has parched up the earth.

It would be a waste of time to even enumerate the theories of malaria, founded on the supposition of an unusual disproportion of the ordinary atmospheric elements, such as an excess or deficiency of oxygen or nitrogen, or carbonic acid, or water. Nor would it be of more use to cite the electrical and magnetic theories of disease, since no analysis of malarious atmospheres has revealed any defect of its elements or of its imponderable constituents. Not a fact sustains any of these opinions, and observations extensively made thoroughly falsify them.* Whatever of change from such causes is observable in malarious places, must be ascribed to their power to excite, not to predispose.

The only theoretic view of malaria to which I incline, is that which refers marsh fevers, and some of the epidemic diseases, to a living organic cause, capable of reproduction by germs, as is alleged of contagious diseases;

* M. Peltier, by constant observations, found the clouds in 1835 almost always positive, in 1836 generally neutral or negative, yet no marked difference in health was observed in those years.

Since these lectures were written, Sir James Murray has defended with much ability, the electrical theory of malarious and epidemic diseases.— (*Lancet, Oct.* 1848.)

but unlike the latter in this, that the germs are not reproduced by the organism of the sick, but exteriorly to, and
independently of, the human body.   In other words, that
as the germs of contagious diseases are reproduced *in*
the body, the germs productive of malarious and other
non-contagious diseases are elaborated and re-elaborated
out of the body, and independently of its agency.   One
is the product of *person*, the other of *place*.   This notion
is sustained by the fact that organic azotized substances
are the only things detected in marsh air or dew, which
can possibly affect the health injuriously.

Although I approve of the reference of malarious diseases to the causation by organic germs, I am far from
being satisfied with the animalcular direction taken by all
who have elaborated a theory on this foundation.   Hitherto it has been so feebly sustained by proofs, as to have
at no time received general favor from the profession,
although supported by some eminent men in almost every
period of medical history.   The chief objections to the
animalcular theory are: 1st. That it has never been shown
that animalcules are poisonous in any way.   2d. That
none of the difficulties of this puzzling subject are thus removed.   3d. That the assumption is hypothetical at first,
and does not in the progress of an examination become at
any time more demonstratively probable, or logically
acceptable.   4th. But the strongest objection is founded
on the superior probability of *the vegetable branch of the
organic theory*, by which I hope to show that very much
of the obscurity of this subject may be dissipated.   This
last objection will, as we advance, rise into more remarkable prominency.

It is painful to be thus compelled to abandon the ingenious theories of our fathers, built up so elaborately and so

industriously ; to brush away the whole labor of the lives of many eminent men, and to reflect upon the time and talent lavished wastefully upon mere day-dreams. We cannot also fail to perceive the great fallibility of human opinion, as thus exemplified, nor can we avoid the dread that we ourselves may have to mourn hereafter, over the unproductive labors of our own lives, or leave to our children the thankless office of removing our worthless mental rubbish, to make way for perhaps not more substantial edifices. Be this as it may, we derive from the review the useful lesson of philosophic humility, which teaches us to state or receive new doctrines with becoming hesitation, and to bring them into *practical* application with prudent caution, and then only when sustained by the prolonged observation of many persons in many places, and at various times.

LECTURE II.

THE CHARACTER, GROWTH, MINUTENESS, DIFFUSION, ALTERA-
TION BY CLIMATE, AND AUTUMNAL PROFUSION OF THE
FUNGI.

In offering to your attention and consideration a theory of malaria, I profess to do no more than present a review of the phenomena which seem to render it probable, without supposing, that, on so difficult and important a subject, I can produce, in your minds, the thorough conviction, which, nothing short of a positive demonstration, could bring home to my own. Not thoroughly convinced myself, I can only be excused for occupying your time, by the belief that the theory I am about to offer, is not only very plausible, but is associated with agreeable and useful collateral inquiries. If we should not discover at the end of our journey, the truth, the search after which has lured us to the path of observation, we shall enjoy, at least, beautiful scenery by the way, and sometimes pluck a flower, and sometimes find a gem.

Standing, at St. George's, in Delaware, more than twenty years ago, upon the bottom of what had been, a short time before, a mill-dam, I found around me the un-decayed stumps of trees which had been, for one hundred and seventeen years, submerged in fresh water. Two or three years thereafter, I again visited the spot, and saw that these stumps, no longer wet, but damp, had been entirely disintegrated by the dry rot, and that they crumbled in the handling. In the handful of dust which I picked up, I found innumerable spores of what I supposed to be Polyporus Destructor, and Merulius Vastator, cryptogamous plants, whose active existence had been bought at the expense of the old stumps. In a moment I conceived that, perhaps, the miasm, so much dreaded in that place, might be, *directly* or *indirectly*, the product of these urgers on of a more rapid decomposition. It was a loose thought at the time; but it gave me a disposition to collect the phenomena which might prove or disprove the agency in the generation of malaria, of living, not of dead plants.

A part of my collection I now offer you. In doing so, I shall present only the affirmative side of the question, believing that no one else is likely immediately to sustain so revolutionary an opinion, whilst professional emulation, habitual prejudice, and even love of truth, will subject it to a sufficiently rigorous opposition. You have, therefore, due notice of the guarded manner in which you are to receive my *ex parte* observations, a notice which I cheerfully give, for I have much confidence in the force of my subject, and do not love my theory well enough to wish its establishment at the expense of truth or reason. Take it, then, for what I may show to be its worth.

Just on the line which faintly marks the division between the animal and vegetable kingdoms, lie the *lichens*, the *algæ* and the *fungi*. These cryptogamous plants are so closely allied to each other, as to be indistinctly separated by naturalists; some of whom include under one division, species which are found differently disposed of by other phytologists. Lindley, following the great con-

tinental cryptogamists, admits that the location, rather
than the structure of these plants, affords a final distinction, and that, while the lichens live on dry and scanty
soils, and algæ in water, salt or fresh, the fungi occupy
the intermediate place, *loving a damp and unsound or
loaded atmosphere*, and feeding on organized matter, the
vitality of which is gone, or going.

In all of them, the element is a very minute cell, not
often distinguishable when isolated, from the elementary
cells of, even animal organisms. Indeed, some of the confervæ, obviously vegetable in one state of existence, as
the *arthrodieæ*, offer in another, the plainest character of
animal life; supposing that animal life is to be inferred
from motions indicating a well-marked power of volition.
Some of the *oscillarias* have an oscillatory movement extremely active and perceptible, and the *ulva labyrinthi-
formis* and *anabaina*, with all the other conditions of a
vegetable, have, according to Vauquelin and Chaptal, all
the chemical characters of an animal. We have, therefore, chemically constituted plants with animal motions
and volition; and those of animal composition, with the
exclusive habitudes and structure of vegetables.

All plants are liable to curious and often great alterations by climate, soil, and season; but the dubious beings
I am now describing, undergo such astonishing modifications, even by the slightest causes, as to perplex, by their
morphology, the sagacity of the best informed naturalists.
They, at least the simplest of them, seem to have so little
inherent tendency to the assumption of form and nutrition, as to take their shape and products almost exclusively from the hand of accident. "One might call it,"
says Lindley, "a provisional creation, waiting to be organized, and then assuming different forms, according to

the nature of the corpuscles, which penetrate it, or are developed among it."

For these reasons, the lowest of the vegetable groups, the fungi, are, in the opinion of some naturalists, equally distinct from plants and animals, mere fortuitous developments of vegeto-animal matter, called into varied action by special conditions, or by combinations of heat, light, and moisture, and capable of existing and of being propagated, under circumstances apparently the most contrasted.

Of all vegetable substances the fungi are the most highly animalized. Like animals, they disengage carbonic acid and imbibe a quantity of oxygen; nay, some of them extricate hydrogen, and even nitrogen. Their chemical composition also allies them to animal structures. They yield the vegetable products, resin, sugar, gum, fungic acid, and a number of saline compounds; but they also afford the adipocire, albumen, and osmazome of the animal kingdom. The basis of these plants is fungin, a tasteless but highly nutritious substance, white, soft, and doughy. It yields, by nitric acid, nitrogen, hydrocyanic, oxalic, and some other acids, and fatty substances, like wax, tallow, and, in some instances, oil.

Of the cryptogamous plants, the *fungi* are distinguished for their *diffusion and number*, for their *poisonous properties, and their peculiar season of growth*, for *the minuteness of their spores*, and for *their love of darkness and tainted soils, and heavy atmospheres*. While, then, I shall present their claims to be considered as the *principal cause* of fevers, I do not mean to exclude the occasional agency of other cryptogamous vegetables; and beg, when using the convenient word *fungus*, to be understood as not entirely denying the agencies of cognate beings of

4

kindred subdivisions, which are hardly distinguishable from it.

Here and there among writers, ancient and modern, a hint is thrown out, that, possibly, plants of the lowest orders may cause malarious fevers; and in some countries, as Spain, for example, even the populace believe that the fungi cause fevers. For, to the practice of eating mushrooms at a sickly season, the Estramadurans ascribed the febrile diseases by which the British army suffered so severely.

A treatise was published at Vienna, in 1775, by J. S. Michael Leger, " concerning the mildew, considered as the principal cause of epidemic disease among the cattle, &c." " The mildew producing the disease is that which dries and burns the grass and leaves. It falls usually in the morning, *particularly after a thunder storm.* Its poisonous quality, which does not continue above twenty-four hours, never operates but when it is swallowed immediately after its falling."

" Should the too bold notion of Nees Von Eisenbeck, that fungi of the most minute forms have their origin in the higher regions of air, and, descending to the earth, produce spots and stains, be confirmed, these *signacula* would have a much more important connection with epidemics than can be otherwise conceded to them."—Hecker, p. 205.

Müller thinks (*Archives,* 1841), that if vegetable cells were to be *seminia morborum,* they could scarcely be microscopically distinguished from the primordial formative cells of our own tissues.

The theory, therefore, which I now offer, is not entirely new. Nay, the learned microscopists, who are making, on the nature and action of elementary cells, such im-

mense contributions to our STORE OF FACTS, not only pre-
pare us for such a theoretic step, but actually, by pregnant
allusions, lead the way. It is, then, not so much a rash
generalization, in advance of the opinion and knowledge
of the age, as a very natural result of that knowledge
collected and classified. It is an expression, if not of the
sentiment, at least of the *science* of the present era.

Under this impression, I undertake the adventurous
duty of developing a theoretic result, not expecting to do
more than obtain for it, at present, a hearing and an examination, since its demonstration, if ever completed,
must exact, for years, the enlightened and patient toils of
many philosophers. "There never is," says Bischoff,
"an important and comprehensive discovery made at once;
the elements of it are generally obtained from different
quarters, and from all these truth at last results."

Imitating the natural philosophers, I have constructed
a theory, not to be esteemed devoutly true, but as, in the
present state of knowledge, the most perfect explanation
of the known phenomena of the case; and as the least
exposed to the many objections easily brought against any
other hypothesis.

It may be thought that the cause assigned is not adequate to the rapid production of the effect. Can a minute vegetable, however distributed, contaminate the air
of a large marsh or field, in the course of a few minutes
or hours? When we remember how minute a quantity
of a reproductive organic virus is, in other cases, necessary to the infection of a proper subject, we might leave
the argument to that defence alone; but I think there is
a better one, in the wonderful growth and ready diffusion
of the plants to whose nocturnal potency I am inclined to
ascribe malarious fevers.

A mushroom growth is proverbial in every language. In a single night, under favorable circumstances, leather, or moist vegetable matter, may be completely covered with mould. Of the more minute fungi, some species pass through their whole existence in a few minutes, from the invisible spore to the perfect plant. Lind says, that the first rains in Guinea have been known to make the leather of shoes quite *mouldy* and rotten in forty-eight hours; showing that the plants which disorganize the leather must have drawn their nutrition, even from its heart, in that time, and, by many successive generations, extended themselves over its total surface. Mr. Berkeley describes a *Polyporus squamosus* which, in three weeks, acquired a circumference of seven feet five inches, and a weight of thirty-four pounds. The *Polyporus frondosus* described by John Bapt. Porta, sometimes transcends a weight of twelve pounds in a few days.

The *Bovista giganteum*, on the authority of Carpenter, the eminent physiologist, has been known to increase in a *single night*, from a mere point to the size of a large gourd, estimated to contain four thousand seven hundred millions of cells; a number which, when counted at the rapid rate of 300 per minute, or five per second, would take the whole time of one person, *night and day, for three hundred years*. A square mile contains upwards of 3,000,000 square yards, or 27,000,000 square feet, so that a single *Bovista giganteum* may present, at evening, an almost invisible single cell, and yet place before morning, nearly 1,800 such cells in every square foot of a square mile.

Notwithstanding the wondrous productions of a *single* individual of one *species*, Fries, the Swedish naturalist, observed not less than *two thousand species*, within the compass of a square *furlong.* The same author tells us, that he has counted above 10,000,000 of sporules in a single individual of the *Reticularia maxima,* so minute as to look like smoke as they rose in the air.

Webster, when writing of the malignant fever of 1795, informs us that *sound potatoes from market* perished in his cellar, in thirty-six hours; and we know now how they perished. It was a parasitic death.

In the *Philosophical Transactions,* Lond. (vol. iv. p. 308, Abridg.), it is stated, that a green *mould* attacked a split melon, and took three hours to sprout, and six to ripen and produce, and let fall new seeds.

At New York, the pestilential season of 1798, Webster says, that he saw a cotton garment covered with dark gray-colored spots of *mildew in a single night,* and that such events were then and there common.

I might multiply examples of the rapid growth and extensive diffusion of fungi, which, like the lowest classes of animals, seem to have a power of development and propagation inversely as their magnitude. The more minute the plants, the more rapid their multiplication; until, as they descend to those of the smallest scale, a microscope shows them in even visible growth. Nothing astonishes one more than to see in the bottom of a watch glass a drop of yeast swelling up, as the *torula cerevisiæ* unfolds itself, and exhibits a forest of fungi, where but a few minutes before, only a spore or two were visible.

"The family of the funguses," says Badham, "is immense. Merely catalogued and described, there are sufficient to fill an octavo volume of four hundred pages of close print, of British species alone. Altogether there cannot be less than five thousand recognized species at present known, and each year adds new ones to the list.

For the single mushroom that we eat, how many hundreds there be that prey upon us in return. To enumerate but a few and those of the microscopic kinds (there are some which the arms could scarcely embrace); the mucor mucedo that spawns upon our dried preserves; the *ascophora mucedo* that makes our bread mouldy; the *uredo segetum*, that burns Ceres out of her corn-fields; the *uredo rubigo*, whose rust is still more destructive; and the *puccinia graminis*, whose voracity sets corn-laws and farmers at defience, are all funguses. So is the gray *monilia* that rots, and then fattens upon our fruits; and the *mucor herbariorum*, that destroys the careful gleanings of the pains-taking botanist. When our beer becomes mothery, the mother of that mischief is a fungus. If pickles acquire a bad taste, if ketchup turns ropy and putrefies, funguses have a finger in it all! Their reign stops not here; they prey upon each other; they even select their victims! There is the *myrothecium viride*, which will only grow upon dry agarics. The *mucor chrysospermus* attacks the flesh of a particular *Boletus;* the *sclerotium cornutum* which visits some other moist mushrooms in decay. There are some *xylomas* that will spot the leaves of the maple, and some, those of the willow, exclusively. The naked seeds of some are found burrowing between the opposite surfaces of leaves; some love the neighborhood of burned stubble, and charred wood; some visit the sculptor in his studio. The *racodium* of the low cellar festoons its ceilings, shags its walls, and keeps our wines in bonds, while the *geastrum* has been found suspended on the very highest pinnacle of St. Paul's. The close cavities of nuts afford concealment to some species; others like leeches stick to the bulbs of plants and suck them dry; these pick timber to pieces, as men pick oakum; nor do they confine their selective ravages to plants alone; they attach themselves to animal structures and destroy animal life; the *oxygena equina* has a particular fancy for the hoofs of horses, and for the horns of cattle, sticking to these alone; the belly of a tropical fly is liable, *in autumn*, to break out into vegetable tufts of fungous growth; and the caterpillar to carry about a *clavaria* larger than himself. The fungous disease called *muscardine* destroys many silkworms, and the vegetating wasp, of which everybody has heard, is only another mysterious blending of vegetable with insect-life. Funguses visit the wards of our hospitals and grow out of the products of surgical diseases. Where then are they not to be found? Do they not abound like Pharaoh's plagues everywhere? Is not their name legion, and their province, ubiquity?"

An ingenious friend proposes as an objection to my theory, that as malarious fevers are specifically the same everywhere, and as the plants of temperate differ totally from those of tropical, regions, how are we to account for their identity? The intermittent is a native of Russia and Sweden, while it is also an endemic of the coast of Guinea, and of the banks of the *Orinoco*.

The answer given is, that of all plants of the same species, only the fungi are known to be natural inhabitants of the various climates of the earth; for to use the words of Mr. Roques, " *we find mushrooms in every climate.*" We saw on a piece of damp leather, at the Cape of Good Hope, the same *mucor mucedo* that penetrates its tissue at Sierra Leone, or St. Petersburgh. Like man, the fungi generally live in any climate, though there are among them some that infest only the steppes of Tartary, and others that revel solely on the sands of *Zahara*. *This ubiquity is one of their most peculiar qualities.*

But why is it, then, if the same fungi create diseases in
Lapland and Senegal, that there is so fatal a difference in
the intensity of them at these two places? As the fungi
of a poisonous character possess acrid and narcotic properties, it is scarcely necessary to consistency to presume
that the same species are everywhere the cause of malarious fevers. Yet, if that were an imperative supposition,
it would not embarrass the question materially, because
naturalists affirm, that *the poisonous cryptogami are rendered yet more poisonous by increased temperature and
moisture*. The amanita muscaria, only narcotic or intoxicating in Siberia, and used there for the purpose of agreeable exhilaration, is mainly irritating in France and Italy,
and therefore, there, a very deadly poison to the mucous
surface and nervous system.

We have an analogous example of the poison-enforcing
power of climate in the fact, that the common hemp evolves
a strong narcotic, in the tropics, while no such excretion
is thrown out from it in temperate regions. In the Crimea,
the *conium maculatum* is used as an esculent vegetable.
The tendency to cause moulds so intensely expressed in
hot climates is seconded by the aggravation of their activity when produced. It is curious too, that tropical
regions excite only the more minute forms in a greater
degree, which according to many writers are most poisonous. "Those that are most injurious, are generally of the
microscopic kinds."—(Badham.) If too, the excess of rain
may make poisonous, in our climate, even the esculent
mushrooms, what may we not expect from the influence
exerted upon the noxious fungi by the prolonged and
heavy rains of the tropics!

May we not find a difficulty in believing that the sporules of the fungi are absorbable into the circulation?

Their volume, or the selective appetency of the mouths of the absorbents and the lacteals, or of the pores of the venous radicles, may offer insuperable impediments to their entrance. The chyle globules are about two-thirds of the size of blood globules in man, and they are supposed to be readily absorbed by the lacteals. Fries states that he has seen cryptogamous sporules of the size of $\frac{1}{10,000}$ths of an inch, which would give them a volume one-third of that of blood globules, and two-thirds only of that of chyle globules. In examining, when mixed together, blood globules and the spori of various minute fungi, I have often seen the latter, in line along the disk of the former, when it required fourteen of them to subtend its long diameter. They were, therefore, at least ten times as small as the chyle-globules. So much for *size*. As to the selective power of the lacteals, we know that they suffer very many and various poisons to pass into the circulation, and that, in this respect, they are much less particular than our fathers imagined. Besides this, we know that fungous growths, both in man and the lower animals, have been found in places, to which their germs could have gained access only by the circulation, or by imbibition. There is, therefore, no good reason for doubting that the spores of fungi find their way to the channels of the circulation, as do the cells of exanthematous diseases, and the virus of syphilis.

The cause of the uniform excess of malarious diseases at the end of summer and in autumn has been an interesting subject of discussion and wonder. Boot, in his life of Armstrong, observes that, "*the most remarkable circumstance* connected with the diseases supposed to arise from malaria, is their general prevalence *in autumn, in every country where they occur.*" Even the yellow fever of places

in which it is an ordinary endemic, is not an exception to
this law, for Baron Humboldt says that, at Vera Cruz,
where "May and June are hotter than September and October, the latter months greatly exceed the former in the
number and vigor of the fevers."*

If mere vegetable decomposition were the cause of such
fevers, we should find them most active in May and
June, when, after the previous autumnal death, and the
disintegrating effects of winter frosts, or soaking rains, the
warmth and moisture of spring and early summer rapidly
decompose the softened textures, to feed the tender spon-
gioles of the swelling vegetation. The great chemists, heat,
light, and moisture, are then most active; and the dead
relics of the former year, prepared by *time, frost* and *rain*,
are ready for the process of decomposition, as the electrical and vital agencies of the countless and thread-like
radices open up their intendered store-houses of nutrition.
Although, therefore, almost every one has supposed that
the autumn is the season of the greatest decomposition,
that process is really conducted in the spring and early
summer *with a tenfold energy*, as may be easily recognized by the extraordinary smell of the earth after a shower
at this season.

Malarious diseases, therefore, are not probably the effect
of ordinary vegetable decomposition; for they occur most
when that is not at, or near to, its *maximum*.

Everywhere they abound, when the general vegetation
has just passed through its great orgasm. But there

---

* The regular return and continuance of this fever in the months of
July, August and September, every year, more or less since its first appearance in these Islands —(Jas. Clark, Dominica.)

Yellow Fever is most active in September, when the temperature has
fallen *much below* that of July and August.—(Wm. Currie.)

is another and special vegetation, *which, whatever may be the climate, has its spring time and summer in the autumnal season* of the year. On the exhausted *debris*, and the varied *exuviæ* of plants, weeds and grasses ; from root to leaf ; under ground and above ground ; feeds a race of vegetables which wait for *their* food to the latest period of the season of heat, and then flourish most when the more perfect forms have completed their annual task, and submit to the inroads of these Goths of phytology.

Governed in a great measure by the phenomena immediately around him, an observer, seeing the period of sickness succeeding to the active vegetative season, assigns the cause to the climatic events which then ordinarily arise. Thus African writers believe that the rains are the immediate producers of malaria, for they descend in torrents in July, when the vegetation of that torrid clime is on the decline. On the other hand, the Sardinian supposes that the sickness of his *hot* and *dry autumn*, is the result of the heat and aridity, and that droughts after rains, and not rains after droughts, cause his *miasmata*.

In the *insular* West Indies, there are heavy rains in August and September, which are sickly months; whereas, the pestilential season of Demarara is also in August and September, although they are there the dry months.

Egypt, although placed in the northern hemisphere, enjoys a climate almost the reverse of that of other countries similarly situated. During the summer scarcely any rain descends. At Cairo there are but four or five showers in a year, and in Upper Egypt only one or two. Near the sea, showers are not quite so rare. Everything, therefore, is, in the hot months, brown and dry and hard—dews rarely descend, and the parched land lies locked up in a barren drought. About the first of June the Nile begins to rise rapidly. Its channel becomes full early in the month, and, at the summer solstice, it pours its waters over its usual barriers. The country is covered with water during the hot summer and autumn, and there is no vegetation, and no disease.

At the winter solstice, the spring time of Egypt begins, and while nature leaps into amazing activity, the husbandman enters on his annual labor of sowing and planting. Towards the end of January, oranges and citrons blossom, and the sugar cane is cut down. In February all the fields are verdant: the sowing of rice begins, the first barley crop is harvested, and cabbages, cucumbers and melons ripen. The sickly season of Egypt should, therefore, on my view, commence in the winter or spring, and accordingly, here as elsewhere, the ravages of disease follow the decline of active vegetation, and *the plague begins*. In 1834, the deaths by plague in December were 109; January, 1835, 151; February, 821; *March*, 4329; April, 1897; May, 321; June, 41 cases. About St. John's day, the country being covered with water, the plague ceases.

We see, then, that *the insalubrity of a place has the most constant relation to the habits of the living vegetation.* Whatever may be the temperature or humidity, the most unhealthy period of the year is, in any given locality, that when the phanerogamous vegetation has completed its annual task of growth, and flowering, and fruitage, and feels the weakness of an exhausting effort, and when to triumph as it were over a worn out foe, the cryptogamous plants plunder and destroy it.

A reference to books, whose authors did not perhaps even dream of this theory of fever, shows, that *the fungi are active chiefly in the end of summer and in autumn.* Dr. Badham observes, that, "A wet *autumn* is generally found to be exceedingly prolific in these plants." This in England, but in Italy the very scenery is beautified by the number, variety, and coloring of these vegetables. "Well may their *sudden apparition* surprise us, for not ten days since, the waters were all out, and only three or four nights back peals of thunder rattled against the casements; and now, behold the meadows, by natural magic, studded with countless fairy rings of every diameter, formed of such species as grow upon the ground, while the chestnut and the oak are teeming with a new class of fruits, that had no previous blossoming, many of which had *already attained their full growth.*" "These are the fungus tribe, a new class of objects which have sprung up suddenly and now beset our path on every side, beautiful as the fairest flowers, and more useful than most of the fruits." "The extremely limited time during which funguses are to be found, their fragility, their *infinite diversity*, their ephemeral existence, these too add to the interest of an *autumnal* walk." "In such rambles he will see what I have, *this autumn*, myself witnessed, whole hundred weights of rich wholesome diet rotting under trees; woods teeming with food, and not one hand to gather it."

Merat and Lens say: "It is usually in *autumn* that they (fungi) are developed in humid places, where the air is thick and unwholesome, with a rapidity that has passed into a proverb."

In the *Cyclop. Amer.* we learn that the best time for gathering mushrooms is *August and September*, and Miller's *Horticultural Dictionary* remarks that *September* is the chief season of their growth.

In the beautiful work of Mons. J. Roques, on the poisonous and edible fungi, is the following language: "*We*

5

find mushrooms in every climate. A very large propor-
tion of them is met with *only towards the end of summer
and in autumn.* Heavy rains, and unseasonably early
heat, may force them in May or June; but they are then
never so perfect. Thunder-storms with rain, develop them
prodigiously."

Of one hundred and five species of fungi treated of by
M. Roques, only one grows at all seasons; four in spring;
one in spring and autumn; five at the very end of summer; eight exclusively in summer; twenty-eight in summer and autumn; and sixty-two exclusively in autumn.
Of the one hundred and five, therefore, ninety-two are
active in autumn, and thirty-six in summer.

Were this essay not necessarily very long, it would not
be uninteresting to inquire, in how marked a degree the
proportion of diseases to seasons, corresponds with that of
the above table: but most of you know already that the
relation is remarkable enough, since the growth of the
fungi and of malarious fevers is generally in the order directly of autumn—summer—spring—winter.

LECTURE III.

THE FUNGI ARE ACTIVE ALMOST EXCLUSIVELY AT NIGHT, AND ABOUND DURING THE PREVALENCE OF EPIDEMICS AND EPIZOOTICS.

THE most common Malarious diseases are not producible by exposure in sickly places, *during the day time.* Whatever may be their cause, it seems to have activity almost solely at night. *Darkness* appears to be essential to either its existence or its power. As this position is not generally acknowledged, I may be pardoned for going into some detail on it.

Dr. James Lind cites the following case.—The Phœnix sloop-of-war of forty guns, was employed in 1766 on the coast of Africa; where also was the Hound on the same duty. Both vessels, after a healthful cruise, put into the African island of St. Thomas, notorious for its pestilential character. Here, of the crew of the Phœnix, slept on shore, seven officers and servants, while three midshipmen, five seamen, and one boy, were also employed on a watering party, which detained them on land at night. Of these sixteen persons, only two survived the malignant fever which followed. The remainder of the crew of two hundred and eighty men, were permitted to go ashore in the *day time*, where the men rambled about at pleasure, followed field sports, and washed their soiled clothing. *Not one of these was attacked with any kind of fever*, and before her return home, the ship lost only one man, and he died of the effects of a blow on the head. The crew of the other vessel, the Hound, were permitted to visit the shore only in the day time, although no other restriction seems to have been laid on them. *Of these, not one died of fever.*

Another equally remarkable case is given by Lind. In 1766, some French Protestants settled in a paludal part of Florida, where finally most of them perished. On some business, they were visited by eight gentlemen, more healthfully seated at a considerable distance, who spent one night there. On the following day, seven other persons from the same place, paid them a visit; but left their district before night-fall. Of the first party, every one was attacked with intermittent fever, and two died; while of the other party, not one individual suffered in the slightest degree.

The judicious Dr. Hunter, of Jamaica, relates cases of nocturnal damage of the same character. In one instance, out of sixty or seventy men sent ashore to water, not an individual escaped fever, while the rest of the crew enjoyed good health.

Doctor James Johnson, in treating of this subject, remarks that, while cruising or at anchor between Batavia and Malacca, his crew lost but one man by fever, who had not spent the night ashore; whereas, almost every one who slept even a single night at Edam, died. No ill effects were experienced from going on shore in the day time. Even *being awake during the night when on land, did not protect the seamen from danger.**

Tratter (*Med. Naut.* i. 456), says, when speaking of

---

* I do not find this remark endorsed by any other writer, but my eloquent friend, Prof. Dickson, confirmed it to me in a recent conversation on the subject.

the danger of exposure to the land-air at night, "every man who slept ashore died, and the rest of the ship's company remained remarkably healthy."

On the authority of Surgeon Allen, we learn, that at Zanzibar, *all* who slept on board ship, escaped; *every victim* seen or heard of, had passed at least *one night on shore.* The captain and forty men from a French corvette, who passed a night on land, were attacked by the coast fever, and not one survived.

Doctor Evans, writing from the unhealthy island of *St. Lucia*, observes, that during the day, "the sportsman wades through the stagnant waters and mangrove bushes, which cover the surface of West India fens, with comparative impunity; but long before the sun has disappeared, he places himself beyond the reach of their poisonous effluvia."

Mr. Webb, Inspector of Hospitals, stated before a committee of the British House of Commons, that the men who remained on board the ships in the noxious climate of Walcheren, were *extremely healthy, although they went ashore to bathe and exercise daily, but never remained on land at night.* Yet it was in that very place that the English army, encamped or lodged on shore, was almost annihilated by malignant intermittents.

Robert Armstrong says, that of the crew of the ship of war Monarch, employed to collect at Xanthus, specimens of ancient art, the large body of men employed on shore were, without exception, attacked with remittent fever, and twenty-four of them died; whilst those who remained on board of the ship were, to a man, exempted from fever.

The inhabitants of our southern country are fully aware of the important truth I have just illustrated, for they avoid as a deadly poison, the night air of malarious regions, but visit them and travel through them fearlessly, during the day time. The precincts of the city of Charleston are especially pestilential, and the country fever, as it is called, is remarkably fatal to the residents of towns and of the upper country. To sleep one night in this district, puts in peril the life of the unacclimated; but no one believes that the most prolonged visit by day is attended with any danger.

In Major Tulloch's masterly report on the health of the military and naval service, he observes that, " the sickness of the shore very rarely extends to the shipping, *though only a few hundred yards from the land.* The visits of sailors to the shore *by day*, did not produce disease. In the Ceylon service, the mortality of the marine force by fever, was 3 in 1000, of the military, 24.6,—or more than eight times as great.

The frigate Potomac, on a three years' cruise, visited some of the most insalubrious stations of tropical regions, and yet lost only 26 men, of whom not one died of fever. Dr. Foltz accounts for this happy exemption from malarious diseases, by stating that his men were never permitted to remain ashore during the night.

During *three voyages into tropical regions,* I always advised the adherence to the safe rule of compelling the seamen to return to the ship at night; and although we watered in places notorious for their insalubrity, and eminently destructive to parties which ventured to remain ashore at night, we did not lose one man by fevers of any kind. In some of these places, the water was stagnant and irritating at first, and caused inflammation of the skin of the legs of the waterers. The heavy odour of the rank vegetation, and the damp feel of the air among shallow pools, where myriads of insects sported, gave lively evidence of a pestilential locality. Besides that, the sickly and bloated looks of the white inhabitants of some of these places, evinced the presence of active malaria.

In vain do we search in the works on received theories, for the cause of this curious influence of night. It is in the day time that evaporation goes on most rapidly, and that chemical changes produced both by heat and light, are in most active operation. The water is warmer, the common vegetation more vivid, and the great chemist, the sun, is urging on the processes of the laboratory of nature. This is of course admitted by many writers, some of whom confess manfully the difficulty of this part of their subject, while others suppose that the miasm evolved during the day, descends at night. Were this really so, it would scarcely account for the extraordinary difference of disease-producing power, between the night and the day; but when we consider how currents of air must sweep away the diurnal emanations, and how late in the night it is before the earth becomes cool enough to detain its proximate atmosphere, we can with difficulty admit this mode of explanation.

It has been also said that the baneful effect is due to the great change of temperature which follows the advent of night, by which moisture is precipitated by the air, and the human frame is chilled and sickened. As there is in the most unhealthy regions (coast of Africa), the slightest diurnal change, as rocky islets (De Loss in Africa), are sometimes most pestilential: as a wall, a road, or a screen of trees, sometimes separates a bad from a good locality, and as no such meteorological differences appear to explain the vicissitudes of the health of different years, we must reject such causes, except as excitants of the power of some poison yet to be discovered.

But when we observe the extraordinary tendency of

fungous vegetables to develop their power only at night, we detect *another analogy between malaria and the fungi.* In vain do we search in the latter part of a day for young mushrooms. The early riser finds them in their prime and abundance. A field which at evening exhibited not a single plant, is often whitened by their little umbrellas in the morning. "It is well known," writes Comstock, "that this tribe of plants springs up almost everywhere, especially among decaying substances, and that *thousands* may be seen in the *morning*, where none existed the evening before."

Even the more durable kinds of fungi appear to add during the day little to their bulk, preferring to grow almost solely under the eye of night; so that these anomalous vegetables not only choose for their growth *the season of vegetable repose*, but *the hours of vegetable* SLEEP. In another respect they are beings of contrast, for, while other vegetables are adding oxygen to the air from which they have extracted its carbon, these, as if they were averse to agreeing with phenogamous plants in any respect, are eliminating carbonic acid, having extracted from the undecomposed organic matter on which they live, its more peculiar animal elements, the hydrogen and nitrogen.

Mr. Sowerby, the best of authorities on this subject, took the minute unopened *volva* of a *Phallus Inodorus* into the house in the evening, and found it in the morning a full grown plant. In his experiments nothing occurred to show that this fungus grows in the day time.

Supposing that the minutest fungi possess the general properties of the class to which they belong, we may readily perceive what prodigious influence must be exerted on them by the damp rich air of a swamp—and if they have, as Heusinger alleges, a polarizing membrane, and consequently electrical relations to the polarized vesicles of a marsh mist, that mist, imbued with moisture, enriched by the terrestrial exhalations, and screened by the shadows of night, may form the most fruitful floating soil for the invisible cells of microscopic *cryptogami:*—so that from the damp earth or the nebulous air, or both, may come out to propagate disease, the cells of an anomalous vegetation.

But it may be reasonably objected, that if these things do grow at night, they should, sometimes at least, taint the day-air of their vicinity, from which they can scarcely be entirely eliminated by an absorbing earth or a dissipating mist. It might be enough to say that, if they have electrical relations to the mist, or ascend only during the night, the quantity necessary to produce morbid results may not remain during the day, but the study of the habitudes of the fungi has revealed *other* reasons for the diurnal changes of salubrity in malarious regions.

In the first place, let me say, that no other vegetables are so strictly limited as these, as to existence or properties, by apparently slight changes in their relations to extrinsics, and yet their germs resist causes of destruction of the most active nature. Boiling water, many of the acids and caustic ammonia fail to destroy them, and they sustain the cold of solid carbonic acid* (Cagniard de la Tour) without the abatement of their productive power.

Dutrochet found that by slightly acidulating a weak solution of the albumen of an egg, various *monilia* were produced, but that when it was made alkaline the genus *Botrytis* appeared. On a neutral or simple solution, no fungi showed themselves.

The *torula cerevisiæ*, or yeast plant, grows in one form

---

* Minus 118° F.

in a saccharine solution containing yeast, and in another very dissimilar shape in stale beer. "There are some (fungi) which are seen only once or twice in an age, and that in places where it is very difficult to account for their formation."—(*Art. Mushr.*—Rees.)

According to Pereira, "the fungi consist of cells and fibres, always sprouting from organized and generally decayed or decaying substances, *not perfected when entirely immersed in water.*"

Fungi (on the authority of Merat et.Lens), appear susceptible of remarkable diversification, according to climate, season, and soil, which *polymorphia* makes their study difficult.

Almost every mineral, however poisonous, supports a peculiar cryptogamous vegetation. Thus we have *hydrocrocis arsenici* in solutions of arsenic, *hyd. barytica* in solutions of baryta. Fungi grow in ink, in wine, indeed, in everything; and naturalists are yet in doubt whether these seemingly diverse things owe their differences to soil, water, and temperature, or to different germs, each capable of growing only in its restricted field.

Some fungi are confined to particular plants, both above and beneath the surface of the ground, and some, as the entophytes, exist only in the *interior* of living vegetables. Even within hard, dried wood, a fungus creates a species of fermentation, by which moisture is evolved. The fungus appears, finally, at the surface, and the ligneous fibre crumbles to dust. It is dry rot; and the destroyers are the *Polyporus destructor* and the *Merulius lacrymans*, and *Vastator*.

Most writers on this subject, including Christison and Foderé, believe that the climate alone greatly alters the fungi; so that some, which are *generally* eaten with safety, become poisonous, and some of the poisonous kinds become esculent. The Ag. Piperatus, according to Haller, is poisonous in France, but esculent in Russia. The Amanita Muscaria, an intoxicating food in Siberia, becomes a deadly poison in the south of Europe. Foderé states, that the most delightful of the esculent mushrooms of France *become unsafe after prolonged rains*. The same thing occurs in South Carolina, where, in very wet weather, it becomes necessary to remove the mushrooms, or keep up the hogs, that they may not be poisoned by that which, in common weather, is eaten to advantage.

As the power of growth, and the quality of the fungi, are so dependent on slight causes, we can scarcely wonder that a plant of this class may be noxious as produced at night, and hurtless as developed by day. Even if produced alike in both, the poison of the cryptogami is so subtle and fugacious, that a little daylight or sunshine may totally alter its properties. Foderé (*Méd. Legal*) tells us that most fungi become safe *when they have been dried*, which Christison thinks probable, as their poisonous properties appear to depend on a volatile principle. Finally, Letellier assures us, that the acrid principle of the agarics is so very fugacious, that it disappears on boiling, or drying, or by maceration in weak acids, alkalies, or alcohol. If, after all this, we find a malarious poison active at night, and not by day, it does not present an objection to the theory proposed, but affords some support to it, since we know of no *other* things which are so materially affected by light and heat.

I am now, gentlemen, about to show you a very curious part of this singular subject, the extraordinary association of fungous life with the existence and propagation of great epidemics and intense endemics. Not only are common moulds more common on such occasions, but there often appear new, or unusual productions of this kind. Hecker and Webster abound with examples of this truth. These moulds were chiefly red, but sometimes *white*, yellow, gray, or even black. They arose in an incredibly short time, on the roofs of houses, on the pavements of cities; on clothes, on the veils, and handkerchiefs of women; on various wooden domestic utensils, and on the meats in the larder. Even the depths of cellars, and the inmost recesses of cupboards and chests were invaded by a blood-like mould, which filled the observers with disgust and horror.

Joseph Mather Smith remarks, " that pestilence; a strong tendency in dead animal and vegetable substances to rapid decomposition; morbid and immature fruits; and a vast amount of insect life; seem to have a common cause in epidemic meteoration." Admitting the extraordinary tendency to decomposition manifested in epidemic periods, Craigie observes, " that the rapid decomposition of vegetable and animal matters is to be regarded, not as a cause of fevers, but an effect of the febriferous state of the atmosphere, which thus displayed its insalubrious influence, not only on the human race, but on the vegetable world, and on *dead animal and vegetable matter.*"

Plutarch, in his life of Romulus, says, that in the first great plague at Rome, it seemed to "*rain blood.*"

On the 3d of July, 1529, when the continental sweating sickness prevailed, a *blood rain*, as it was termed, appeared at Cremona. In the sweating sickness of the English, there was remarked " an exuberance of the lowest cryptogamous vegetation."

In that calamitous period, which commenced An. Dom.

250, Decius being emperor, a pestilence began, which cut off, in the next fifteen years, half the human race. Eusebius relates that the air was so impure, as to "cast a *mould* like *turbid dew*, of a cadaverous hue, *on every object.*" Cadenus likened it to *the gore* or *blood* of the dead.

In 1813, at Malta, on the 14th of March, "the light showers that fell in some parts of the island, brought down a *reddish earth* with them. The same phenomena were observed at Palermo on the same day. In April, the plague commenced its ravages in Malta. (Maclean.)

Boyle makes the observation that, at Naples, in 1660, there was a pestilence, during which, curious mould spots appeared on garments. So, in the plague of 746, spots, in the form of crosses, were observed on clothes.

At Brussels, in 1502, a pestilence drove the people from the city. On their return, they observed that, in that single season, a cryptogamous vegetation had covered the roofs of the houses. (Webster.)

At New York, in 1795, Bailey describes the destructive influence of that sickly season on cabbages, different kinds of fruit, &c. "It was remarkable that cherries did not come to perfection, and very soon showed *a disposition to decay*. The apples began to fall nearly a month before the usual time. *Those which came to maturity could not be kept so long as it is common for them to be preserved.*"

Webster also speaks of that year, (1795,) as peculiarly fungiferous. To use his own words, "the air of New York produced astonishing effects in the way of mould." Garments were spotted in a single night, the pavements became mouldy, and wooden furniture and utensils were spotted. Even desks, carefully closed, were invaded by mildew.

The year 1798 was remarkable for its prolonged heat

6

and drought. Looking over the distinct and simple daily narrative of Dr. S. P. Griffitts, I find no mention of rain from the 20th July to the 4th September; and other writers describe this season as peculiarly hot and dry. Notwithstanding this, Condie and Folwell inform us, that *" the different kinds of mushrooms were found in great abundance during their season."* Webster also states, that in this year there were *fogs which had a singular odor*, and "even the pavements were covered with a mouldy dew." Through Dr. Rush, we also learn that the great heat of the season brought peaches to perfection nearly three weeks before the usual time; whilst apples, after being gathered, rotted much sooner than is commonly observed.

In 1799, at New York, similar phenomena were observed; and Webster noticed the extraordinary death of multitudes of flies, which became *white exteriorly*. This disease seems analogous to that of the muscardine of the silkworm.

In pestilential Africa, when the rains and the sickness commence together, the fungiferous powers are fearfully developed. According to Park and Lind, the first rains *stain the clothes*, and make even woolens and leather *mouldy* and rotten in a day or two.

In St. Lucia, the most unhealthy station of the West Indies, "during the driest period of the year, a pair of boots are covered with vegetation, within twenty-four hours after being cleaned." (Evans.) In confined places, in unhealthy stations, the air is of a mouldy odor, " *earthy and mouldy.*" (Robt. Armstrong.)

During the epidemics of yellow fever at Natchez in both 1823 and 1825, Cartwright noticed an extraordinary tendency to the production of mould, so that the shoemakers complained of the extreme difficulty of preserving even new articles in their line. Cartwright was surprised at this, because, the meteorological state of the atmosphere would not account for it. *It was a fungiferous power irrespective of unusual dampness.*

During the prevalence of the cholera in Philadelphia in 1832, I was shown in several different places a splendid vermilion colored *mucor,* which attached itself to paste, starch and other vegetable preparations. The housekeepers who noticed it then, had not observed it previously, nor have any of them seen it since. At that time, the flies died as in New York in 1799, and were covered with a whitish dust. Confirmatory of these observations is the assertion of Copplez, Lamoth, and Coulin, that alimentary substances putrefied with unusual rapidity in the season of cholera.

In a letter addressed to me on the 3d of December, 1847, by Josiah G. Cable, M.D., of the U. S. service, I am informed, that, at Monterey, in a season always excessively dry, and then peculiarly so, under a burning sun, and on a lofty range of country, the men suffered greatly from miasmatic disorders. He also remarked the uncommon fungiferous tendencies of the place, as manifested by the mould on fruit, and the cacti, and aloe, and even "when a dead Mexican was turned over on the battle-field, his clothes were found to be covered *with a white fungus.*"

In fine, the history of epidemics abounds everywhere in examples of the cryptogamous luxuriancy of epidemic seasons. It is noticed by the careless observers of the middle ages, in more than half the recorded cases; and the ancients speak, not unfrequently, of offensive fogs and frightful mists and moulds. The spirit of the mist,

according to Hecker, stinking and pestilential, moved
over the face of devoted England, where, as it went, were
scattered the seeds of the *sudor anglicanus*, by which that
kingdom was almost depopulated, and sometimes the people of the villages were entirely exterminated.   Many
epidemics, as cholera and plague, select for peculiar residence and ravage, damp, dark, noisome places, where
want of light and dryness and ventilation, must especially
favor fungiferous processes.   The instinctive aversion to
mouldiness, as to serpents, seems to be, therefore, not
without its utility, and in seeking the elevation in society
which gives to man cleanly habits and an airy residence, individuals find a physical exemption from disease and pain
even more valuable than the social enjoyments.

In the history of epizootics, are related a multitude of
examples of the production of destructive diseases, apparently brought upon cattle and other animals by mould.

The fatal *angina maligna* of cattle, a gangrenous disease, which prevailed in 1682, was attended by a *blue mist*
or dew on the herbage of pastures.

The milzbrand, *a gangrenous* disease of cattle, not unusual in France and Germany, is, according to Thomasin,
very prevalent in Burgundy and Provence, where it affects
the herds chiefly of low and humid districts in *summer* or
autumn after inundations, by which the pasturage is de-
teriorated and the fodder *moulded* and *mildewed*.   The
disease thus acquired by cattle, may be conveyed to other
animals including man, by ingestion (Chaussier, &c.) or
even contact with the skin (Morand, Duhamel, Thomasin),
producing in either way symptoms of fever in some persons,
and malignant pustules in others.   Sometimes a gangrenous
fever is the consequence, and at other times only a local
gangrene of a very intractable character ensues.   That the

poison upon which this very curious disease depends, is vegetable, may be strongly inferred from the fact that its *virus* is capable of resisting, not only the heat of boiling water, but the action of caustic lime prolonged for at least two weeks. (Gruby.) No animal substance or even ovum, is known to have the power of resisting such agents, while, according to Cagniard de la Tour, the spori of the fungi can withstand means of destruction quite as potent. And, on the authority of many authors, we know that "unlike most seeds, they (the spori of the fungi) seem capable of resisting the prolonged heat of boiling water, infused in which, and poured upon the ground, they are still capable of producing, each after its kind." (Badham.) So tenacious of its integrity and power is the *virus* of malignant pustule, that it can retain its destructive properties even when the wool or hair has been cleansed and woven into cloth, or the hide converted into leather. (Bayer.)

In this instance we have a disease originating in a grazing animal, probably from its food, when mildewed, which disease may be propagated by inoculation or ingestion, and of which the germs resist the heat of boiling water, the caustic action of lime, the detergents of the washer and weaver, and the prolonged tanning of the leather-dresser. Nothing known to us but the spores or nucleoli of the fungi are capable of accounting for these phenomena. Vimat, a commissioner of the Royal Academy of Medicine, made a report to his constituents, on an epidemic which occurred in the department of La Muerthe near Marsal, which began in the cattle fed on recently inundated swamps. It was a *carbunculous* affection, which *without material change of character*, affected subsequently the inhabitants of the same district. (Fourcroy, *Med. Eclairée.*)

6*

J. S. Michael Leger, published at Vienna, in 1775, a treatise concerning the *mildew* as the principal cause of epidemic disease among cattle. The mildew is that which *burns and dries* the grass and leaves. It is observed early in the morning, *particularly after thunder-storms.* Its poisonous quality, which does not last above twenty-four hours, never operates but when it is swallowed immediately after its falling.

There is, in the wild regions of our own western country, a disease called the *milk-sickness,* the *trembles,* the *tires,* the *slows,* the *stiff-joints,* the *puking fever,* &c. Of this curious malady, I have already, gentlemen, given you in its proper place, an elaborate history; but it may not be useless here, to recapitulate the leading thoughts of that lecture.

An animal affected by the cause alluded to, usually exhibits the symptoms of the disease upon being driven hard for a very short distance, perhaps only a hundred yards.* It then trembles, loses its regular power of locomotion, staggers, falls, makes ineffectual attempts to rise, becomes convulsed, and dies. When the affection arrives under quietude, the animal seems to lose its voluntary route, and strays irregularly and apparently without motive. Its power of attention is impaired, the eyes become red and turgid, and the color deepens from a bright to a dark red. Finally, it trembles, staggers and dies. When other animals—men, dogs, cats, poultry, crows, buzzards and hogs— drink the milk or eat the flesh of a diseased cow, they suffer in a somewhat different manner. The attack in men

---

* This reminds us of the tetanode state of a frog, which being affected by a small dose of strychnia, falls into convulsions at the touch even of a feather. Marshall Hall recognizes the resemblance in this, to a diseased predisposition, waiting for an exciting cause.

is usually ushered in by nausea, followed by vomiting, which at irregular intervals recurs, until the close of the case in death or convalescence, a period usually of from four or five to ten days. In the first stage of the attack, the sufferer complains of severe pains in the limbs, but chiefly in the calves of the legs, and sometimes at the nape of the neck. A headache is a common event. Even before the open attack, during the incubative period, constipation is observed, and a very obstinate torpidity of the bowels is a marked feature during the whole case. The abdomen is commonly enlarged, and doughy, and presents a very singular, diffused pulsation, most conspicuous to the right of the navel. In some cases there is gastric or abdominal pain and tenderness, in others, even the prolonged vomiting does not cause pain; but usually there is perceived a curious and *intense sense of heat* at the *epigastrium*, which produces a desire for cool drinks, independently of a sense of thirst.

As in most intense fevers, the pulse is often in this one, even natural, or, while the face is flushed, the extremities become frightfully cold, and the pulse falls to preternatural slowness or is accelerated to one hundred and ten or one hundred and twenty per minute. (Buck.) In some cases no sensorial disturbance is perceived, in others there is intense nervousness, extending sometimes to delirium, vigilance, coma. Such cases commonly prove fatal, after the occurrence of *singultus, subsultus,* a hurried irregular pulse, cold extremities and a sunken countenance.* There is, according to every detailed account, a singular fetidity of the breath, not like any smell known to the describers;

* Sometimes the *hair,* cuticle and *nails* drop off. (Lea.)
M. Roulin tells us that in Colombia, the maize is liable to a kind of fungus or ergot, which occasions the loss of nails and hair.

which, with obstinate vomiting and costiveness, peculiar, soft enlargement of the tongue, and an abdominal pulsation, most distinctly felt *to the right of the umbilicus*, constitute the marked distinctions of this malady.

The animals made sick by the beef of the first one, have been, in their turn, the cause of a like affection in others; so that three or four have thus fallen victims successively.

Whatever the poison may be, it resisted the influence of the cook, in all the customary modes of preparation, also the action of diluted acids, and alkaline solutions, and chlorine, and some of the chlorides. *Infusion of galls* alone seemed to abate, but not to destroy its virulence. The water, in which poisoned beef had been boiled, acquired no poisonous properties; while the beef remained as noxious as ever. Butter from diseased cows, heated until it caught fire, did not lose its deleterious properties. (Graaf.) The urine of diseased animals, collected and reduced by evaporation, produced the characteristic symptoms. Milk of affected cows, or sluts, was very poisonous to their own young as well as to other animals, whilst the lactation preserved themselves from the malady, so long as they were milked regularly.

The animals originally affected, are only such as live upon herbage, such as cows, horses, goats, and sheep. The pastures in which the disease is found, are *always* the unbroken soil of the new country. The action of the plough, even for a single season, is regarded by most authors as a *permanent* corrective.

Whatever may be the poison, its most potent activity exists in the end of summer and in autumn, chiefly in September and October. One writer denies the truth of this statement, but a large number assert it very positively.

It also acts only *at night*, or until the dew has been exhaled from the grass in the morning; for even the worst ranges are safe during the day, except where they lie in thickly wooded districts.

This disease has been found in rich alluvial places, on high barren ridges, on open plains, and in the deepest woods. Its place is sometimes confined to a small space inclosed as a "sugar-orchard," and entirely destitute of water; while it extends in other cases throughout a long narrow range of country, for as much as one hundred miles.

From the testimony of authors, each of whom has a peculiar opinion on the point, milk-sickness may prevail in wet or dry, hot or cool autumns, the character of the season seeming to have no especial relation to the severity of the epizootic.

The period of incubation varies in cattle, from two to ten days, when an attack is not sooner excited by violent exercise. When the disease is produced by the swallowing of poisonous beef, or milk, butter or cheese, the nausea and vomiting may occur almost instantaneously, or may not appear until after the lapse of several hours or even days.

Whatever may be the poison, it seems, according to the experiments of Graaf, to be reproductive within the system of the poisoned animals; for, the quantity of flesh necessary to produce the diseased effect, was about the same, whether taken from an animal originally affected, or from others successively poisoned by its flesh or milk.

Most writers say, that attempts to inoculate with the blood, milk, &c., of affected animals have failed, but Drake asserts, on the authority of two credible witnesses, that the milk-sickness was produced in them by skinning diseased cows.

The autopsy showed gastro-intestinal inflammation, enlargement and softening of the liver and spleen. The meninges and brain exhibited congestion, inflammation, serum, lymph, pus. In all the fatal cases, *the blood failed to coagulate*, and there was uniformly a contraction of the stomach and intestines.

Authors generally admit, that only the grazing animals take the disease originally, and that other animals can only receive it through the medium of their flesh, or milk, after they have been poisoned. As all animals seem impressible, there is a fair inference against the aerial character of the cause of milk-sickness, by which, if it exist, they should be equally and originally tainted. The facility of the correction by the plough, the insoluble and non-volatile nature of the poison, evinced by the effects of boiling or roasting the beef, and of the evaporation of urine even to dryness, all show clearly that the poison is not atmospheric, not aëriform or vaporous. It seems, therefore, plain enough that cattle receive it into the stomach as *food* or *beverage*. That the poison is not found in the water taken by the grazing animals, seems highly probable, because it has not been found subsequently to be soluble in that *menstruum*, or, indeed, in any other simple liquid, whilst the truth of this position has been almost demonstrated by confining them in limited enclosures, where, notwithstanding the total absence of water, many of them have, in repeated instances, exhibited veritable symptoms of the trembles. A critical examination of the waters of infected regions has failed to show peculiar or poisonous properties, and the plough corrects the evil, without being shown to be able to alter the waters materially.

It seems, then, very probable, that the poison, whatever it may be, is swallowed with the food. Now the food is more or less soiled with earth. It is, also, in its most hazardous condition, covered with dew, and is infected by insects, and the seeds of various plants and flowers.

Of these, the soil cannot give the venom, as it would not lose such a power by the action of the plough. A mineral poison would also be easily detected in it, and could not propagate itself through a succession of animals; nor has it a reproductive power.

We are reduced, therefore, to the only remaining hypothesis, the introduction of an *organic poison* of some kind, animal or vegetable, into the nostrils or stomachs, (probably the latter,) of the affected animals. The long latent continuance of the poison in the body, the apparently small quantity of it necessary to create disease, and the seeming reproduction after reception, all enforce the conviction that the virus is *organic*.

Having rendered probable the presence, in these cases, of an organic agent, the usual course of medical reasoning would lead us to assume its *animal* derivation, especially as it seems to have, even in the system, a reproductive power. But just at this point of time, the microscopic discovery of the frequent connection of vegetations with cutaneous and mucous diseases, and the probability that, in other, and somewhat analogous cases, cryptogamous plants exercise a disease-creating power, embarrass us with a new element of difficulty.

Animal poisons are usually soluble, are commonly innocuous in the stomach, are not most potent at night, do not affect particularly the autumnal season; nor can we see how the plough could correct the evil, if of an animal character. The extraordinary fixity and indestructibility of the germs of this disease, point strongly to a vegetable source.

We are thrown back, therefore, by a kind of necessity, on its vegetable origin, and among vegetables we find none, whose habitudes and modes of action, so strongly as the fungi, entitle them to the sad distinction of creating this singular malady. They grow in autumn, they grow at night, they are disarmed by light and heat, they have extraordinary tenacity of life and texture, and yet are repressed by very slight alterations of soil and circumstance. They are usually poisonous, and produce curious and diversified maladies. Women are less affected than men by their poison, and children escape more readily than men and women. Some of them, after sending their poison through the system, escape unchanged by some one of the emunctories, as the *amanita muscaria*, by the kidneys. As we are reasoning upon probabilities here, let me ask what animal poison, what mineral poison, offers so many and so strong analogies, to entitle us to esteem it a cause of the milk-sickness.

LECTURE IV.

MOST OF THE FUNGI ARE POISONOUS, AND PRODUCE DIS-
EASES RESEMBLING MARSH FEVERS.

NOT only are the fungi generally, poisonous to a singular degree, but the phenomena attendant upon their
introduction into the system are so peculiar, as to arrest
the attention both of the toxicologist and pathologist. In
most cases, the poison lies dormant, for a time after its
ingestion, then excites a morbid action of a febrile character, continued in some instances, remittent or intermittent in others, which is sometimes followed by abscesses
or gangrene, as observed in typhoid fever and plague,
occasionally by locked jaw and yellow skin, as in yellow fever. Even when using habitually, fungous food
of a slowly poisonous quality, such as rye affected with
ergotætia abortifaciens, females of adult age, and *the
richer classes of society* are, to a remarkable degree, exempted from the disease-producing potency, which exerts
itself so disastrously in some parts of France and Swit-
zerland, on the poorer and more exposed portion of society.

Of late years, too, it has been found that many cutaneous disorders, and at least one mucous disease, are, if
not absolutely dependent on, at least closely associated
with, and aggravated by, the growth of minute cryptogami. That these predatory fungi are really causers of

7

the maladies with which they are uniformly connected, is made still more probable by the demonstration of the existence in insects, and even many larger animals, of *contagious cryptogamous diseases, which, transferred from animals to plants, and from plants to animals*, become very destructive, not only to their immediate victims, but to important commercial interests dependent on them.

It is scarcely necessary to prove to any intelligent reader, that the fungi are commonly poisonous. The caution with which mushrooms are bought, and examined, and cooked, evinces a sufficient knowledge everywhere, of the danger of eating the wild kinds. But as I am elaborating an argument upon a new and difficult subject, a few quotations, to show the sentiment of the best informed persons, may not be inexpedient. "By far the greater part of the tribe," says Comstock, "are poisonous. Some of them are so exceedingly virulent, as to destroy life in a short time. Adepts, therefore, in botany, dread the wild kinds." "So poisonous," says the author of the article mushroom, in *Rees' Cyclopedia*, "is one species of agaric, as to kill the very flies as they settle on it. The *Agaricus muscarius* is therefore used to poison flies and bed-bugs. Burnett quotes several curious cases where death has arisen in persons who have eaten mouldy (fungiferous) bread, mouldy pork, mouldy cheese, mouldy ham, pie, &c.

But it is rather to the *peculiarities* of these poisonings, than to the general fact, that I would direct your attention. The first of these is the production of FEVER. Pereira tells us, "that the symptoms produced by poisonous fungi, are those of *gastro-intestinal irritation, and a disordered state of the nervous system*," a not inexact general definition of a malarious fever. "In the human system it (Agaricus muscarius) produces *shivering*, followed by that kind of *delirium which attends an ardent fever.*"—(*Rees' Cycl.*, Art. Mushr.)

A careful examination of the diseased potatoes of the British isles, from which that kingdom has of late suffered so much, shows the uniform existence in them, of "the fibres of a fungus called *botrytis*, from its grapelike form, or of one called *uredo tuberosum*, which may be observed ramifying round the cells which enclose the starchy corpuscules. Now these plants, however minute, are not self-generated, but must be produced by some seminal impregnation, transported by the atmosphere, and peculiarly adapted to fructify upon the *Sol. Tub.* This vegetable distemper, like *that of the cholera*, while general in its diffusion, is determined to particular localities and plants, by predisposing causes; yet it is not always dependent on these, having occurred in many regions where such causes did not materially operate."—(Ure.) "The effects of using diseased potatoes, were in the first stage rigors, heat of skin, quick pulse, and abdominal pain; in the second stage, rose colored spots, migratory and evanescent, and diarrhœa; in the third *stadium*, a tumefaction of the muscles of the neck, shoulders and arms, acute pain there, and in the worst cases, erysipelas of the face and scalp, and œdema of the eyelids."—(O'Brien.)

The effects of heavy single doses of ERGOT are, first, anorexia, nausea, vomiting, dryness of the throat, and thirst; secondly, abdominal pain and tumefaction, and diarrhœa; thirdly, weight and pain of head, giddiness, delirium, dilated pupil, somnolency, coma; fourthly, disturbed circulation by *increased fullness and frequency*, or *feebleness and slowness of the pulse*. *Formication* is a not infrequent consequence, while protracted use creates, not only febrile symptoms, but, as in malignant fevers, *a disposition to gangrene.* Christison describes the effects of its prolonged use, as *weariness and formication.* "IN A FEW DAYS *fever sets in,* with a *hemorrhagic tendency, rending pains of the limbs,* and at length, *dry gangrene of the fingers, toes,* or even *legs,* which drop off by the joints." In some cases, the author just quoted reports *contraction of the spleen** and enlargement of the liver, as among the effects of ergot.

Dodart, who acted under a commission of the French Academy of Medicine, reported to that body, that ergot occasioned *"nervous phenomena and malignant fever, with stupor."*

In 1826, Dr. Westerhoff saw two children who had been poisoned by mouldy bread; their faces were *red and swollen,* excited and haggard, tongue dry, inextinguishable thirst, feeble and frequent pulse, abdominal pain, vomiting and purging, vertigo, headache, great depression of mind and body, mental indifference, and somnolency.

On the 10th of June, 1839, at a musical festival at Aldenfingen, about six hundred people ate various kinds of meat, which, after being cooked, had been kept *in a badly ventilated cellar for nearly three days.* Upwards of four hundred of them were, *within ten days,* attacked by nausea, vomiting, some mental disturbance, colic pains, tenderness of the epigastrium and diarrhœa. In the progress of the cases, disturbed circulation, constipation, fetid evacuations and tympanitis allied the cases to typhoid fever, *and nine died of this fever.* An autopsy revealed inflammation or ulceration in the lower part of the *ileum.* Those who did not go to the festival, but partook of these cold meats at home, suffered in a similar manner; whilst

* The spleen is sometimes lessened.—*Art. Typhus, Dic. de Médecine.*

those at the festival who dined on bread and cheese, escaped all disorder.

Diseased wheat (*Phil. Trans.*, Lond. 1762,) produced at Wattisham, a sickness with sphacelation. Seven persons of one family suffered the loss of one or more of their limbs, and one had a blackness of two fingers, but recovered.

The febrile disease from the use of rye is, according to Thompson, (*Lect. on Infl.*) most prevalent in *wet* or *moist* seasons, and in thirty-three years, M. Noel met with this malady three or four times, and always in *rainy and moist seasons*. He also says, that among fifty patients, he *did not find one woman;* and he makes the very curious statement, that *only the poor and ill-fed were its victims.*

Pereira describes almost *choleric* effects of the poison of fungi, when he states, that in some cases, the powers of the vascular system were "*remarkably suppressed*, the pulse being *small and feeble*, the *extremities cold*, and the body covered with a *cold sweat.*"

It may not be disadvantageous to insert, in this place, the description of a yellow fever which became epidemic in the U. S. Frigate Macedonian. It was given under oath to a court martial by Surgeon Chase. "There were pains in the head, loins, and limbs, tenderness at the epigastrium and sometimes in the fauces; nausea, vomiting, diarrhœa or constipation; *the face was flushed, and sometimes swollen, the pulse was either frequent and full or slow and small;* the eyes were red and watery, the mind was dejected; and there was, *ab initio*, low delirium or violent madness."

The famous *sweating sickness* usually commenced with a short shivering fit, which, in malignant cases, convulsed even the extremities. Many experienced, at the beginning, a disagreeable creeping sensation, or *formication,* on the hands and feet, which passed into pricking pains, and an exceedingly painful sensation *under the nails.* Some persons were afflicted with swollen hands and feet. In many the countenance was *bloated and livid,* the heart "*trembled and palpitated,*" and lividness and rapid decomposition evinced the tendency to sphacelation. *The plague,* with its symptoms, its abscesses, and its mortification, might be taken for a case of fungous poisoning in its more intense forms.

You may now, gentlemen, turn to another curious effect of the poison by the fungi: I mean, *periodicity.* Many authors mention, among the phenomena, *intermittency,* or *remittency.* The most singular of such cases is cited by Christison, who tells us that a whole family, consisting of a woman and her four children, were attacked by a *tertian fever,* by living exclusively for four months on *edible mushrooms.* The peculiar cause of the fever was made more manifest by the fact, that the husband of the woman, who lived on other fare, escaped all disease; while a *cutaneous eruption and subsequent gangrene of the extremities* attacked finally those who had the fever. Westerhoff observed in those who were poisoned by mouldy food, an *intermittent somnolency,* which he terms a remarkable feature of the case. M. Gassand saw cases of ergotism where the sensations either of heat or cold were *intermittent.*

Several other writers mention this feature. The mental disturbance intermitted in one case, inflamed eyes in another, and all the phenomena in a third. A young woman who ate a dish of *Agaricus clypeatus,* and was attacked with nausea, vomiting, bilious stools, and a frequent pulse, had *a marked remission* on the fourth day. The patient was at ease throughout the night, the skin was moist, and the pulse better. The other symptoms all abated, and the patient slept. On the fifth day, *the symptoms returned*, with delirium, sighing, anxiety, failing pulse, great dyspnœa, *partial yellowness of the skin*, and even a *locked jaw*, as in some cases of yellow fever.

Another author cites a case of fungous toxication, in which " *the remission* was so well marked as to attract attention. The *Dic. des Sci. Méd.* reports cases of this kind, in which occurred *the most acute pains*, which *were intermittent;* and often there was a pause of two or three days, during which the sick could attend to their affairs." A recent epidemic fever in Scotland presented both the yellow skin, and the long and curious intermissions described in the above cases.

A reverend gentleman of the Protestant Episcopal Church, in the city of New York, in the preceding year (1845), went with his family to a place near Sing-Sing, and about three miles from the Hudson, which was selected because of its reputation for health, and its exemption from malarious diseases. In August and September, when mushrooms were very abundant, and when the country people abstained from their use, under the impression that they disposed them to fevers, the clergyman's lady, in her frequent drives, collected them daily, and for some time subsisted almost exclusively on them. The remainder of the family ate them more sparingly, and less frequently. About the end of September, the lady was attacked by an irregular fever, without periodical chills, but marked by an exacerbation on every second day. Thus the nature of the case was not suspected, until the return of an attack in the spring, which became regularly periodical in June, and assumed a distinct tertian form.

It was then cured readily by the sulphate of quinia, and other means approved for intermittents.

In 1844, I busied myself with collecting and examining various species of fungi, most of them of a poisonous quality. For several hours a day, I hung over these specimens, watching the successive growths of fungus superimposed on fungus, and endeavoring, with a microscope, to measure the relative size of their spores and nucleoli. Whilst thus engaged, I was, for the first and only time since my early childhood, attacked by a tertian, and was compelled to resort, after the third paroxysm, to the usual treatment for an intermittent. Whether this attack was the result of the slight vegetable decomposition, or an effect of the inhalation of spores of invisible fungi, I know not, but the coincidence was at least singular. That the latter supposition is the more probable one, is sustained by the well-known fact, that after an evacuation by an emetic or cathartic, of the poisonous fungi, no remedy is so valuable, as a corrective of the febrile and other consequences, as the preparations of cinchona. Merat and Lens, after describing cases of disease produced by fungi, remark, that *preparations of the bark are the best remedy.* Confirmatory of this opinion is the statement of Dr. King, of New York (*New York Med. and Phys. Journ.*, 1825), that, in a case of ergotism, wine and bark constituted the most effective remedial agents.

We thus, see, gentlemen, that when patients are slightly affected by the fungi, symptoms arise which closely ally the cases to those of common marsh fevers; and that the resemblance is still farther improved by the discovery, that both are to be most successfully treated by the antiperiodics.

More intense poisonings, by superadding buboes and *mortification* to other symptoms, bring fungiform diseases into close resemblance to the *plague*. Indeed, when we read first of the course and character of most epidemics, and then turn to the history of *cryptogamism*, in its diversified groupings, we cannot fail to be surprised at the many points of resemblance.

The plague is esteemed by many persons, but an exaggeration of paludal fever. Mirolanoff, among others, inclines to this sentiment, and says that, at Archial, both officers and soldiers, who had intermittent fevers, were attacked with buboes and *carbuncles*. At Adrianople, Dr. Rinx observed that the slighter forms of plague were not distinguishable from intermittent fever, until the appearance of the buboes. Begin and Baudin also concur in the supposition, that plague is of the family of intermittents. John Hunter, M.D. of Jamaica, saw carbuncles in intermittent fever. After some continuance the part mortifies. "I have seen this in the *scrotum*, and also in the foot, and occasionally the loss of a toe." He also enumerates locked jaw as among the incidents of such cases. In 1798 Dr. S. P. Griffitts observed, in one day, two cases of mortification in yellow fever: one around the anus, and the other in a finger. Arujula met with carbunculous cases of yellow fever, and several gangrenous tumors.

The Hungarian fever of 1566, presented a kind of crisis by tubercles on the top of the foot, which, if neglected, ended in mortification, and many suffered amputation. (Skenkius.) In 1600 there raged throughout Europe a *mortal* colic, which usually destroyed life within four days. The patient became almost immediately senseless, *the hair fell from his head*, a livid pustule appeared upon the nose, which consumed it, and the extremities became cold and mortified. (Webster.) M. Roulin relates that in Colombia, the maize is liable to a kind of fungus or ergot, which occasions the *loss of nails and hair.* The poisonous property is lost by conveying it across the Cordilleras. (Merat and Lens.)

Marcellinus tells us that there " arose, in the reign of Marcus Antoninus, a fatal pestilence, which began at the sacking of Seleucia, and extended over the civilized world, from Caledonia to Persia. It was supposed to have arisen *from the foul air from a box,* opened by a soldier, in search of plunder. The symptoms were, *light fever, and a gangrene on the ends of the feet.* In Rome alone, 10,000 died of it daily." The dark, damp old box, the evidence of a reproductive power, and the light fever and severe gangrene, speak strongly in favor of the fungous origin of this epidemic. Something very like this happened at Canton, where three persons were attacked with fever, and two with gangrene, in consequence of breaking unexpectedly into a coffin, long buried. Fortunately, no reproduction took place, and the terrible malady ceased with its first victims.

In another pestilence, A. D. 262, described by St. Cyprian, the patients suffered from despondency, debility, involuntary evacuations, *inflamed mouth, swollen stomach, and sparkling eyes. The disease destroyed the feet, hands, sight, hearing, and organs of generation.*

Chirac thus describes an epidemic at Rochfort, in 1741. Chilliness, great pain in the head, sense of *intoxication,* small pulse, syncope, *epistaxis,* inexpressible loss of strength, constant agitation of the limbs, leaden, cadaverous face, eyes dull or sparkling, continual nausea or vomiting, suppuration of the parotids, buboes, carbuncles, especially on the head and hands.

Gualtier de Claubry abounds in descriptions of gangrenous fevers of a low type. Thus in the typhus at Mayence, in 1813, and 1814, there was "*often gangrene of the extremities.*" At Forgau, in 1813, there was "*often gangrene of the extremities.*" In the hospital at Langres, in 1806, there was sometimes "dry gangrene of the feet." Fouquier, in describing a fever in the department of the Moxelle, in 1813, speaks of partial gangrenes on the surface of the body.

Thouvenel, a physician at Pont a Mousson, describes a febrile gangrene of projecting parts. Roux, Gilbert, Descastaing, Reveille, Parise, Frisal, Boin, Mauguis, Thouvenel, Fleury, Latourette, Robert, Fouquier, Gras, Castel, &c., mention, as events in fever, partial gangrene of the nose, ears, fingers, toes, and the loss even of a whole limb. So also, John Hunter, McGregor, Pringle, Griffitts, Hillary, Deveze, Fellowes, Arejula, and others, describe, as accidents of yellow and other fevers, mortification of the stomach, intestines, lungs, arms, legs, and scrotum.

One of the most striking examples of a gangrenous fever, presented itself in the village of Deerfield, in New England, of which the following account is extracted from the Walpole Observatory, of the 9th Nov., 1807. "On Tuesday, 2d September, 1807, Joshua Fink, an unmarried man, of about 25 years of age, returned from Hartford in Connecticut, to his father's house in Deerfield, where he became very ill, but finally recovered his health. On the 25th, twenty-three days after his return, his mother, Amy Fink, and his niece, who had nursed him in his illness, were attacked with *chilliness and vomiting,* followed by *excruciating pains and soreness* throughout their whole frames. They both died within twenty-four hours, *in a putrefactive state.* In that family circle, thirteen or fourteen persons were similarly affected, and only three or four recovered. Most of them died within twenty-four hours, in *a putrid state.* On the 7th of October, Sally Blacker was taken ill of the same disease and died on the fifth day." The narrative declares that she did not putrefy immediately like the others, EXCEPT ONE OF HER FINGERS.

While poisonous fungi create the usual signs of fever, affecting the mucous tissue of the *primæ viæ* with inflammation, congesting the brain, disordering the liver and spleen, disturbing the circulation, and lessening or vitiating all the secretions, they produce, when used to excess, or for a prolonged period of time, a marked tendency to the ulceration and sloughing of compressed parts, as in typhoid fever, or to the mortification of the intestines or extremities, as in yellow fever, epidemic, camp, jail, or hospital fever, or to carbuncular destruction, as in plague. Every fungus of a poisonous nature does not produce all these morbid phenomena ; but even the most nutritive of the mushrooms will, when long and almost exclusively eaten, manifest *the characteristic effects of the class.* In sudden poisonings, the peculiar tendency to sphacelation does not often occur, and when a disease is occasioned by only one or two doses, we seldom meet with gangrenous phenomena ; but dreadful mortification often follows their slow and protracted application. As far as I can obtain information, it is made apparent that the more minute fungous forms have the most poisonous and gangrenous influence. Thus the long use of bread made of diseased rye (Ergotætia abortifaciens) causes, not only a distinctly formed fever of a remittent character, but gangrenous sloughs in the intestines, and the dry rot of the extremities. We can scarcely resist the conclusion that this last effect is the consequence of the absorption and vital action of the fungous spores in the parts thus destroyed. Vegetables furnish us with many analogies. The diseases to which fruits and bulbous and tuberous roots are liable, are often the effect of absorbed fungi. Thus, in the microscopic journal, we learn, that Arthur Hill Hassall caused decay at will, in sound fruit, by inoculating it with the spawn of fungi from rotten specimens. The mere bruising of fruit would not cause decay, unless fungi or their spores were present. So, the dry gangrene of the potato, so fatal of late to that esculent in Germany, and since, in Great Britain and Ireland, is produced by *the absorption and destructive reproduction* of fungous germs in its very substance.* The analogy seems complete; for, in both sets of cases, fungi produce the disease, and in both, a destruction of the life of remote parts is the consequence. In the potato and apple, the result is demonstratively caused by fungi. In the animal, may we not safely infer it, especially as several instances are recorded, where the putrid matter, conveyed to puerperal women by the hand of the surgeon-accoucheur, has appeared to produce gangrenous *phlebitis;* just as was similarly excited, a gangrene of the fruit and the root.†

Even to my own mind, gentlemen, arises the objection, that most of my analogies result from cases in which the poisonous articles were taken into the stomach, and that too, in large doses, such as could not be received into the

* Ann. des Sci. Nat., Sep. 1842. M. De Martius.

† In Simon's Chemistry, published since the first delivery of these lectures, we are told that Scherer obtained in the abdominal cavity of one who died of metroperitonitis, organisms resembling minute algæ.

8

system in any other mode. That objection seems more specious than sound, when we remember that very small doses of poisons are highly effective when inhaled by the organs of respiration. Thus a very few drops of chloroform will, by inhalation, produce effects on the nervous and vascular systems, more potent than can be created by any dose, however great, thrown into the stomach. A drachm of ether inhaled from a bag, will intoxicate, stupefy, and prodigiously excite him whom ten or even twenty times that quantity would not greatly move by the stomach. So, while it requires not less than thirty grains of arsenic (Christison) to kill an adult, I have known nearly fatal results from the inhalation of less than half a grain of arseniuretted hydrogen. Now it is obvious that, of the small quantity of the respired articles mentioned, a much smaller quantity is absorbed by the pulmonary membrane, and passes into the circulation. Of the few drops of chloroform used, at least nine-tenths must be exhaled by the breath, and thrown away. But when organized substances find their way into the tide of blood, and that too with vital energies capable of reacting on the elements of the sanguine current, it requires but little acquaintance with physiological and pathological phenomena, to induce us to dread the most fearful results. Even when their vital powers are destroyed by mechanical or chemical processes, vegetable poisons act, in the smallest portions, with great violence. How much strychnia, or digitalia, or aconita is requisite for the disturbance of functions, or the arrest of vital action? Certainly much less than we may readily suppose could be inhaled by a sleeper, if such things were suspended in his atmosphere, even with faint diffusion. But the experiment of Prout during the cholera in London, in 1832, if to be relied on, showed a gain in atmospheric specific weight of one sixty-second part; which would give scarcely less than a drachm by weight of some poison, suspended in each cubic foot of the atmosphere of London. That quantity of air may be inhaled during common respiration, in fifty inspirations; and, as most persons respire not less than fifteen times a minute, a cubic foot of air may pass through the bronchial tubes in three minutes and a half. How much, then, of such a poison, may be presented to the bronchial surface, in the course of a single night! With how much more force, too, will it act, when it assails the system through that channel! Substances presented to the gastro-intestinal surfaces are mixed up with various secretions, mucus, saliva, gastric juice, bile, pancreatic liquor, and special exudations from the peculiar glands of each successive section, while aërial poisons, unmixed and unfettered, are applied at once to a surface on which, behind scarcely a shadow of a film, circulates the blood prepared, by the habitual action of the respiratory function, to absorb almost every vapor, and every odor, which may not be too irritating to pass the gates of the *glottis*. It is, perhaps, for this reason, that we have so instinctive a dislike of mouldy smells, and of humid musty places, and unhappily, we discover, that *in the abodes of filth and poverty, where misery dwells, and moulds do most abound,* the great non-contagious epidemics find and destroy the greatest number of victims, because there is the especial domain of fungiferous potency.

I have hitherto spoken to you of the action of fungi, when swallowed, or when inhaled by the respiratory organs. I am now about to direct your attention to a not less curious department of our subject. I mean the association of obvious fungous growths with the cutaneous and mucous diseases both of men and animals. In the very

time in which we live, there has arisen almost a new science, founded on the discovery that many cutaneous diseases, some maladies of the mucous system, and a number
of the disorders of insects and reptiles, seem to be produced by vegetations in the living tissues, by which comfort is impaired and sometimes life sacrificed.

Caffort alleges, that the *agaricus fimetarius* is found in
ill-conditioned wounds (*Annal. de Montpelier*, 1808), and
Mery and Lemery cite cases where fungi grew on the skins
of animals, even when not wounded or ulcerated. Schoenlein and Remak observed, and Fuchs and Langenback
confirmed the observation, that forms, apparently vegetable, and of a fungiform structure, rooted themselves in
the skin of *porrigo favosa*. Gruby subsequently investigated the subject more fully, and alleged that the *crusts
of porrigo are almost entirely composed of the plants.*
The vegetable nature of the disease seemed to be established by the transfer of it by inoculation *to a phanero-
gamic plant*, thus imparting to a vegetable a disease contagious in man.

Since these striking discoveries have been made, microscopists have detected vegetations in *porrigo lupinosa,
impetigo scrofulosa, serpiginous ulcers, sycosis menti, and
porrigo decalvans.* To the latter, Gruby has given the
name of microsporon andouini, in honor of the able writer
on the muscardine of the silk-worm. We have now to
encounter among the phenomena of disease, porrigophytes,
mentagrophytes, &c. &c. Each disease has its fungus,
perfectly characterized by form, habits, position and propagation. For example, porrigophytes are seated in the
cells of the epidermis, while mentagrophytes reside in
follicles between the hair and the walls of the follicles.
The former have a proper capsule, are very rarely granular

in the stem, and their spores are large and oval, while the latter have no capsule, granules almost always appear in the stem, and the spores are small and round. The former descend into the hair-follicles, the latter ascend from the roots of the hair to the epidermis.

Not alone the skin, but the mucous membrane affords a field for the growth of cryptogamous plants, at the expense of the health of that membrane. In the *Comptes Rendus* for 1842, M. Gruby describes a fungous plant, which seemed to be the cause of the aphthæ which so often annoy sucking children, and are not unfrequently a torment to older persons. So minute is this plant, that each little conical elevation of the milk thrush is composed of a *multitude* of these vegetables, each having its leaflets, branches and sporules. The roots are implanted in the cells of the epithelion, and the spores are not more than the one-ten thousandth of an inch in diameter, or about a third of the diameter, or a ninth of the volume of a blood-globule.[*]

Vogel, in the same year, discovered vegetable *Paras* in the aphthæ, and found their organic covering capable of resisting the action of the water of ammonia and strong acetic acid.

Dr. Berg, a Swedish physician, has since treated this subject more at large, and shown that these aphthous protophytes are propagated not only from mouth to mouth, at the usual temperature of the body, but that they can live, and effect a reproduction out of the body, and at lower temperatures, when placed in contact with substances con-

---

[*] The nucleolus in the cell-germ frequently appears immeasurably small, or even entirely escapes the eye with the highest magnifying power, yet it probably serves as an introduction to the whole formative process.— *Schleiden.*

taining albumen, or any nitrogenous compounds. These Paras are supposed, by Berg, to be active, even after being dried, and he suggests the idea of their transmissibility in this state through the atmosphere.

Dr. Arthur Farre, of London, read to the Microscopical Society a paper on the minute structure of some cryptogamous vegetable, which escaped in a kind of membranous mass from the bowels of a female, who was slightly indisposed before, but who suffered severely for about twelve hours immediately previous to their expulsion. Dr. Farre was not able to refer them to known species, but supposes that *the reproductive spores* may have been swallowed in some beverage, *and become so altered, by receiving supplies from an organized surface,* as to present new and unknown appearances.*

Mr. Goodsir (*Ed. Med. and Surg. Journ.,* vii.) describes curious vegetable organisms developed in the stomach during indigestion.†

Mr. Gruby and Mr. Goodsir, without any concert, at different times and places, detected *transparent nucleated cells* in the glands of Peyer, in a diseased state, from *typhoid fever.* Whether these were animal or vegetable cells could not be determined, but that they were vegetable germs is made probable by the subsequent discovery by Schoenlein and Langenback, of *organized vegetable fungi in the body of a person who had died of typhoid fever.*

Hanover detected a species of leoptomitus agardh on the mucous membrane of the mouth and tongue of *two* typhoid patients, and also in the *bladder* of a young child.

---

* Confervæ, discharged in a case of dysentery, are described by Dr. Bennett.

† More recently, similar instances of this production, termed *sarcina* by Mr. Goodsir, have been noticed in pyrosis, by Mr. Benjamin Bell, and Dr. Wilson.

Rayer found byssoid vegetations *on the pleura* of a tuberculous patient, and *in the intestinal canal* of a case of pneumothorax.*

In 1838, Boehm published the discovery of *vegetable filaments* on the mucous membrane of the intestines of those *who died of* CHOLERA.

Quevenne and Hanover found the yeast plant (*torula* cerevisiæ) in diabetic urine.

The frequent action of the fungi in the production of disease, is made analogically more probable by observing also, how many diseases of the lower classes of animals are obviously dependent on the assaults of the cryptogami. Among the earliest observed and most thoroughly studied of these diseases is that of the *muscardine* of the silk-worm. This curious and costly malady was described for the first time in 1835, by Bassi, of Lodi, and M. Balsano, of Milan. Afterwards, in 1836, M. Andouin, who had devoted much time and attention to the subject, published a work on it, and in honor of the first describer gave to this deadly vegetable-enemy of the silk-worm the name of *botrytis bassiano.* His statement is to the effect that there is found in *decaying* or *mouldy moss*, a very minute fungus which bears very small whitish spores. These, placed near to the silk-worm, attach themselves to its surface, and by some unexplained means, gain access to the pigment, under the cuticle, and to the subcutaneous adipose tissue. They are soon converted to the use of the vegetable; and indeed the acute observer of this subject could mark the transformation of the fatty tissue of the worm into radicles of the cryptogamic vegetation. By degrees the plants

* Scherer, cited by Simon, describes, as being found in the peritoneal cavity, after death by puerperal peritonitis, minute cells, *organisms resembling algæ*, granules and nuclei.

penetrate from within to the surface, where they have their fructification, and *whiten* it with sporules. Thus created, the germs attach themselves to other worms, and *a contagious disease, of vegetable origin*, devastates the cocoonery of the silk-producer.

The most curious part of this case is the capability of a plant to live at the expense of either another vegetable or of the silk-worm. A singular passage in the oldest book in the world carries this idea even beyond modern discovery, which, as often happens, seems to be rapidly approaching to the truth, as announced three thousand years ago. In the 13th and 14th chapters of Leviticus, where the subjects of scall and leprosy are discussed, we find the following singular language:

Chapter xiii.—" The garment also that the plague of leprosy is in, whether it be in the warp or woof of *linen* or *woolen*, whether *in a skin* or any thing made of skin; and if the plague be *greenish or reddish*, in the garment, it is a plague of leprosy, and shall be showed unto the priest, and the priest shall shut up the plague seven days. If the plague be spread in the garment, the plague is a fretting leprosy. He therefore shall burn that garment.

" If the plague be not *spread* in the garment, then the priest shall command that they wash it, and shut it up seven days, and behold if the plague have not changed its color, it is unclean, and if the plague be somewhat dark after the washing, he shall rend it out of the garment, and if it still appear, it is a spreading plague, and then shall burn that wherein the plague is."

Chapter xiv.—" The priest shall command that they empty the *house*, and he shall look if the plague be *in the walls* of the house, with hollow strakes, *greenish* or *reddish*, which in sight are lower than the walls. Then the priest shall shut up the house seven days, and shall look, and behold if the plague be spread in the walls of the house, then the priest shall command to remove the stones, and he shall cause the house to be scraped within round about, and they shall replace them with new stones, and they shall take other mortar and plaster it. And if the plague come again, and break out in the house, then the priest shall come and look, and behold, if the plague be spread in the house, it is a spreading leprosy, and he shall break down the house.   *   *   *   *   *   *

"This is the law for all manner of plague of leprosy and scall, and for the *leprosy of a garment and of a house.*"

There is here described a disease, whose cause must have been of organic growth, capable of living in the human being, and of creating there a foul and painful disease of contagious character, whilst it could also live and reproduce itself in garments of wool, linen, or skins; nay more, it could attach itself to the walls of a house; and there also effect its own reproduction. Animalcules, always capable of choice, would scarcely be found so transferable; and we are therefore justified in supposing, that *green or red fungi, so often seen in epidemic periods,* were the protean disease of man, and his garment, and his house.

Hecker also says, " These spots (signacula), and especially the blood spots (red cryptogami), were seen at a very early period, as, for instance, in the sixth century; and again during *the plagues* of 786 and 959, when it is said to have been remarked, that those on whose clothes they frequently appeared, and seemingly imparted to them a peculiar odor, were more liable than others to an attack of leprosy. Hence thay were named clothes leprosy (*lepra vestium*)."

Continuing my enumeration of the fungous diseases of animals, I cite Ehrenberg as having detected a vegetation, *chætophora meteorica*, growing on the scales of the *salmo eperlanus*, and creating disease. Henle has found vorticellæ on the toes of Tritons, producing *gangrene* and death. Hanover saw another kind of vegetable, which, accidentally attached to dead flies in damp places, could, by inoculation, be communicated even *to water salamanders*. Dr. Stelling, of Cassel, found similar products on frogs, weakened by other experiments; and Valentine tells us that *Achyla prolifera*, a kind of mould, very often attacks animals, preventing the development of the ova of fishes, and rapidly extending from an individual to a group.

M. de Longchamps having occasion, in 1840, to dissect an eider duck (anas molissima) while yet warm, found a mould on the mucous surface of its air tubes. The membrane beneath was diseased, and the spores of the plant were little more than half the size of blood-globules. Rousseau and Serrurier observed a different kind of mould in pigeons and fowls, as well as in the *cervus axis* and *testudo indica*. In a male parroquet, which died tuberculous, a greenish pulverulent mould was found on a false membrane *between the intestines* and *vertebral column*. Moulds in animals are also described by Müller, Retzius, Mayer, Jæger, Heusinger, Thiele, &c.

A *stryx nictea* (water fowl), brought alive from Lapland to Stockholm, died dyspnœal. The lungs and *thoracic cavities* were found to be universally covered with mushroom-like, flat, rounded bodies of a yellow-white color, separable from the mucous membrane without injury to its surface.

A *falco rufus*, in the zoological collection at Berlin,

was examined by Dubois, who found the same white um-
bilicoid bodies, quite fresh, in the air cavities, and also in
the abdominal cavity near the kidneys. Müller, Link,
Klotzsch, and others, declared them to be vegetables.

I fear, gentlemen, that I have wearied you by the citation of so many facts, which, all nearly alike, lose interest by repetition. But, on new ground like this, you
must bear with me, if possible; as it is necessary to show,
by many witnesses, that fungi not only obviously produce
diseases, but that they must be absorbed and carried into
the circulation, as they are frequently found by the best observers in the world, even in the shut sacs of the body.

LECTURE V.

EXPLANATORY CHARACTER OF OUR THEORY—LATENCY—
LIMITATION — DRYING — MOULDY SHEETS — YELLOW
FEVER — CHOLERA — TROPICAL HEALTH — SUCCESSION
OF EPIDEMICS.

A THEORY of malaria should not, in this enlightened
age, be received, which does not, at least plausibly, account for the apparent irregularities, seeming contradictions, and anomalous inconsistencies of the subject, which
now so greatly obscure all the usual modes of explanation.
In this respect I hope to show the very great superiority
of that which, I presume, is, by this time, not unfavoura-
bly viewed by my hearers.   The diffusion of the fungi;
their properties as a class; their acknowledged power of
producing diseases of a febrile character, marked by periodicity; their nocturnal power and autumnal prevalence;
their love of the damp dark places in which febrile epidemics delight; their companionship with epidemics and
epizootics; their obvious association with many cutaneous
and some mucous diseases; their production of some contagious diseases of insects; and the progress of diseases
from cattle, which are sickened by eating mildewed food,
to human beings, sometimes by the use of the flesh, and
sometimes, as in the cases reported by Vimat, by the
simple exaltation of epidemic influence: all these details,
numerous, diversified, and well sustained by authorities,

should, I hope, induce my auditors to advance into the
subject of the present lecture with, at least, some partiality for the new doctrine.

No one has yet attempted to explain satisfactorily the
cause of the latency of the malarious poison. "The
latent residence of narcotic marsh poison in the system,"
says Stevens, "is incredible." Lind says, that a man
may be attacked by fever almost immediately after exposure to its causes, or after a day or two, or even after
weeks. Usually the attack occurs within a few days of
the time of exposure, and often on the following day. It
is not easy to comprehend this, unless we suppose that the
poison received into the system, is organic and vital, and
that the phenomena of disease depend on its modification,
and reactions in the body. In this way we can also understand how such a poison may remain dormant, like some
of the animal poisons, and that its absorbed germs may
be stimulated not only by time but season, following laws
which we are just beginning to study.

This study is, necessarily, very limited as yet, for we
are denied a direct examination, and trust often to analogies, feeble sometimes, and at others scarcely perceptible.
On this part of the subject, as in one already discussed,
we can only examine the effects of visible fungi, when
swallowed, and trust to the light thus imperfectly obtained
for a farther progress. It is, however, a very curious
fact, that, of all the known poisons, that of the fungi lies
dormant in the system for the longest time.

One of the greatest peculiarities (Christison) of fungous poison is, *the interval before attack*, and the *difference
in that interval*. He endeavors to explain both these
phenomena by ascribing them to the difficult solubility of
the poisonous matter, surrounded as it is by vegetable

9

pulp and fibre. But, in the splendid work on mushrooms, by M. Paulet, published in 1812, we are told that the extract and alcoholic tincture, and even the juice of the *agaricus bulbosus* and *vernus,* when given to dogs, did not make them sick in less than *ten hours* after their administration.

Christison mentions the poisoning of six persons by the *Hypophyllum sanguineum* or toad-stool (Puddock-stool), in Scotland, most of whom were attacked, after the lapse of twelve hours, one after twenty hours, one after twenty-four hours, and the last in about *thirty hours.*

Gmelin quotes seventeen cases, which did not exhibit symptoms of toxication until the expiration of *a day and a half* after the meal at which the poison was swallowed.

Corvisart's journal relates, that of some soldiers, who ate of the *agaricus muscaria,* a part were attacked with gastric symptoms almost immediately, but that others were indisposed only after the lapse of more than six hours, of whom four died.

In the *Histoire des Champignons* of J. Roques, we are told that a dog, fed on a *patie* made of the *agaricus venenatus,* exhibited symptoms of uneasiness only after an interval of *ten hours.* The same author relates cases where longer periods of time were necessary to develop the poisonous effects of the *amanita citrina* and the *agaricus maleficus.*

We see, then, that the poison of the fungi may remain apparently inactive for from an hour or two to even a day and a half, and that, too, when swallowed in large quantity. If we were now to look for any known poison as explanatory of the latency of malaria, should we not be inclined to say, that only that of the fungi exhibited, in this respect, a strong analogy? We *know* of no other morbific agent whose action is so uniformly and irregularly postponed.

Nothing more startles the student, who has been taught to believe in marsh or other exhalations as being the grand cause of autumnal diseases, than when told, that often a low wall, a common road, or a screen of trees, can, and does, arrest the progress of marsh miasmata, though the wind from the marsh whistles freely past them, bringing with it even the paludal odor. He is also told by McCulloch, the great advocate of the vegeto-aerial theory, that sometimes agues prevail exclusively on one side of a street, and that *inch by inch, and foot by foot*, the site of the Roman capital is invaded by malarious diseases. The absurdity and inconsistency of these various positions strike at the very root of all the old theories. On the other hand, when we suppose that the poison is a fungous one, *progressively marching over the soil*, sustained by the rich air and pregnant moisture from the marsh, we can readily suppose that the wall, or the road, or the wood, may limit its progress. Besides this, the spores of all fungi are more or less electrical, and are, therefore, likely to be arrested by the trees of a wood.

Authors have admitted that malaria appears to act in many instances as if it could exert no power, except when close to the spot where it originated, whilst in other cases, it seems to be wafted to a great distance from its apparent source. If we suppose the existence of germs susceptible of reproduction, and progressive growth, these seeming contradictions fall at once. The interruption of progress by a road or wall justifies this view of the mode of conveyance, and the many facts which show the narrow limits of the poisonous activity, enforce it strongly. The place, the very spot, where the disease is found, must reproduce the cause of it for itself, and if the conditions of growth are not present, then will the spot be exempt, even if very near to the most poisonous places. Thus may we, and only thus, explain the occurrence of agues, yellow fever, and cholera, on only one side of a house, or one end of a room, or one side of a street, or wall, or road. A wind may indeed waft the spores in small quantity to a distance, but unless there are there the conditions essential to an adequate reproduction, the spores must lie dormant and harmless. For such reproduction, the marsh mist may be one of the most important elements, but that alone will not suffice, since we know that the disease is not proportional to its frequency or intensity. Other and very local conditions seem to exercise a peculiar power. Thus a new house is known to resist disease better than an old one, and a residence protected by an annual cultivation, immediately around it, is more safe than one which is encircled by lawns in grass. During some unusually sickly years, when scarcely an inhabitant of the skirts of the city escaped marsh fever, the wind set, often for a long period, directly from the infected regions into the heart of the city. In perhaps half a minute from the time when the south-western air left the meadows and pestilential borders of the town, it had crept into every chamber of the place; yet physicians here, well know that no disease of a malarious character invaded these chambers, which were, most of them, left open during every night of the sultry autumn.

Writers entitled to credit and authority, by position and professional character, assert, that a gauze veil, or a gauze screen in a window, adds much to the security of the wearer or the occupant of a chamber, in even the most unsound places. We can scarcely see how any gas or vapour, simple or compound, could be arrested by such a defence; but it is easy to suppose the detention of organized and comparatively bulky bodies electrical and glutinous, or moist.

However intense may be the virulence of a miasmatic atmosphere, its powers are greatly abated by artificially drying it. Hence, wood-cutters and waterers on the coast of Africa, find it advantageous to kindle a number of fires in the vicinity even of their sultry work. Lind attributed the greater health of the ship Edgar, compared with that of her consort, to the location of her cooking apparatus, "between decks." Folchi, a Roman writer, says, "many persons are known to me who have, during many years, preserved themselves from fever, in the worst parts of the country around Rome, by adopting the most rigid caution in retiring within their houses before evening, closing the windows, *warming the rooms*, and taking care not to go out in the morning until the sun has been some time above the horizon." Old John Kaye speaks of the exemption of cooks and smiths from the sweating sickness. (*Sudor. Angl.*) There is no other poison, save that of the fungi, so far as we know, which is thus disarmed by dryness and heat. In any view of the case, the fact is inexplicable unless we suppose an organic cause, to which the absence of humidity is antagonistic.

Immemorially, the sleeping in damp sheets has been thought hazardous to health; but the keepers of hotels and boarding-houses know that the danger is very slight, unless the sheets have been put away in a damp state, and have acquired a *mouldy* smell. The constant practice of the hydropathists shows the little hazard of a wet sheet, while daily experience demonstrates the certainty of at least stiffened and painful muscles, and an arrest of the

Schneiderian secretions, after spending an hour or two between damp and musty bed-clothes. The Scottish High-
landers are said to dip themselves, dress and all, into the
sea, when obliged to sleep out of doors, after being
drenched by rain. As water is supposed to act unfavour-
ably by means of its coldness, we cannot easily explain
the known benefit of this substitution, except by a reference to the acknowledged power of salt to prevent the
growth of fungi.

It may seem rather curiously nice to notice another
point connected with this part of our subject; but as you
are all students now, and will, I hope, become true scholars
hereafter, I will observe, that every one who searches
for knowledge among old books and manuscripts, has been
occasionally attacked by sternutation, and at least a temporary coryza, when he has disturbed the dust which has
long slumbered within their leaves. As the dust of a
room swept daily, and the pulverulent clouds of a summer
road do not so affect him, he seizes his microscope and
detects the cause of his sufferings, in the numerous organic
spores which have grown into power to torment, among
the dampness and darkness of the leafy envelopes.*

We can scarcely doubt the events recorded by Lind,
Rush, Webster, Hosack, and others, of the partial introduction of yellow fever into places always otherwise exempted from it, by trunks of unwashed clothes, brought
from infected regions. Boerhaave, Cullen, Lind and Rus-
sell think fomites, which are soiled and placed in a confined depository, are more to be dreaded than the excre-
tions of the sick.

---

* My distinguished friend, Professor Hare, finds this experiment among
his old papers, even a hazardous one, as it always seriously affects his
health.

Hosack asserts, that the virus is, under such circumstances, *augmented in quantity.*

Hecker, to whose opinions I have already referred, holds that *fomites may even aggravate the infectious powers of a virus.*

Doctor Rush mentions one trunk-case, in detail, and says that he heard of two other instances, in all of which only those suffered who opened the packages. According to William Stevens of Santa Cruz, " *The poison is made more intense by being confined in clothes and bedding.*"

In 1747, the trunk of a young supercargo who died at Barbadoes, was opened in Philadelphia in the presence of Mr. Powell, Mr. Hatton, three Welshmen, a cooper and a boy of Mr. Powell's: all sickened, and died of yellow fever within a few days.

"I have seen the cases of some servants in Mr. O.'s family, attacked by yellow fever, upon receiving the clothing of a relative who had died of that disease in the West Indies, at a time, too, when no yellow fever prevailed in New York." (Hosack.)

On the same authority, we learn that, after the death by yellow fever of the late Gardiner Baker, whilst on a visit to Boston, where it prevailed epidemically, his clothes were sent home to his wife, then a resident of Long Island. The opening of the trunk was followed by yellow fever, of which Mrs. Baker died. No disease of the kind existed at that time in New York or its vicinity.

A recent report to the Legislature of New York on the subject of Quarantine, contains unanswerable facts of this kind, both numerous and well authenticated. Were yellow fever a contagious disease, these examples of propagation by fomites might be easily explained; but as its non-contagiousness is clearly shown, by even stronger testimony than that above cited in favor of introduction by fomites,

we are left to explain the difficulty, as best we may, con-
sistently with a belief in its importation by trunks and
clothes, and a thorough conviction of its total want of contagious power.   There is left but one escape, and that lies
in the supposition that fungi, when lodged in the trunks
among filth and animal matter, find, in darkness and
dampness, the fittest imaginable growing place.   That, in
scarcely any of these cases, the disease advanced beyond
those who inspected or handled the clothes, is only proof
of the usual difficulty of sowing successfully tropical
seeds in temperate climates, and of the inaptitude of fungi
to grow under any but the nicely adjusted conditions upon
which many of the tribe rely.   Were I disposed to support farther the opinion just defended, I might cite Dr.
John Bard of New York, Dr. Lining of Charleston, the
late Dr. John C. Otto, Drs. Bond, Cadwallader and Gra-
ham of the last century, Dr. Holt of New Orleans, Dr. W.
S. W. Ruschenberger, Dr. Joseph Bailey, Dr. Westerveldt,
Dr. Vaché, and a host of others of the present day for
examples of propagation by trunks and clothes.

Of a similar character is the question of the importation
of yellow fever in ships.   From the angrily mooted case
of the Hanckey, in 1793, by which the yellow fever was
brought from Africa to the island of Grenada, to that of
the Eclair Steamer, which, in 1845, carried it from the
same coast to Buena Vista, and even to England, there has
been a tempestuous dispute about importation and contagion.   The contagionists point to the Bann at ascension,
and even at Bahia, and to the Buck at Bristol, a high and
healthy village on the Delaware, and to the Vanda at the
usually salubrious town of Roundout, one hundred miles up
the North River, as evidence of importation, and, *of course*,
of *contagion*.   They can go even further, and show that there
are at least eighty recorded examples of the production of

yellow fever in unusual places by vessels which came from its ordinary *habitat*.

On the other hand, physicians very generally reject the doctrine of its contagiousness, because it is not carried about by infected persons, because its victims, however much crowded together in a hospital which is removed to a short distance from the infected spot, do not produce it in those who visit or nurse them, or sleep with them at night. Persons thus habitually exposed, show their susceptibility, by suffering an attack by visiting, even for a few minutes, only the open *streets* of the morbific place. This objection is so strong as to throw the contagionists into all kinds of devices to defend their untenable position; such as, conditional contagion, contingent contagion, concurrent local causes, *tertium quids*, between the imported and local agents, all of which, entirely hypothetical, depend for existence, even in the minds of their expounders, upon the first assumption, the contagion of yellow fever; an assumption which owes its acceptability solely to the fact of importation in ships, and propagation by fomites, together with the hitherto insuperable difficulty of giving to it a different explanation. "There is our position!" say they to their opponents; "destroy it if you can!" The opponents are reduced to the necessity of giving to numerous well attested phenomena a flat denial. The anti-contagionists, on the other hand, point to the dispersing invalids of a pestilential city, and ask, why they carry not disease to the country. They exult in the immunity of the hospitals, and, in their turn, inquire with confidence, "Where is your contagion?" They are answered by subtleties, and suppositions, and hypotheses. Is not all this very contrary to the true spirit of philosophy? Would it not be better to admit that yellow fever is often imported in ships, is now and then carried in trunks, and may possibly be sometimes an accident of the locality?   Might it not be also said, that we know of no contagious disease which presents any analogy to the contingent contagion claimed for yellow fever, and that, therefore, we must, for the present, suppose that *it is portable* and yet *is not contagious?*

If I have made a good footing for the fungi, as producers of diseases very like to yellow fever, I may be indulged in *my* hypothesis, which alleges, that a tropical fungus, carried off in dark, damp, animalized holds of ships, or in the offensive clothes of sick or dead seamen, may be introduced into the summer-clime of unaccustomed places, and there, as it came from, may go to, the shore, and be sometimes reproductive.   May I not suppose that the germs, when once ashore, may slowly migrate landwards, and even by chance be carried or wafted to other neighboring spots, where they may grow, and create new *foci* of disease? that the requirements of an exotic may make such visitations rare, and such dispersions unusual? and that the equatorial plants may be nipped, and even totally destroyed by an unaccustomed frost?

Through this theory of ours, we can easily see why the disease may be imported, why it is imported rarely, and why it makes so slow a progress from the spot to which originally brought.   It will, also, explain its non-contagious character, and even its occasional but rare visit to a village or hamlet.   It may also account for its apparently spontaneous appearance in such places as Charleston, Savannah and New Orleans, in which the winter may not be severe enough to kill the germs, but yet may so affect them as to make their reaction difficult or partial.

It is only thus that we can comprehend how a *perfectly*

healthy crew may bring with them, in the closed hold of their ship, the germs of disease, which, after their dismissal, may pestilentially affect the "stevedores" who discharge her, or only the laborers *who disturb her ballast.*

We can thus, too, explain the *usual pause* between the first set of cases caught by visitors to, or laborers on board, the ship, and the attack upon the inhabitants of the vicinity. This curious interval, noticed by almost every writer, occupies about ten to fifteen days, whilst the period of incubation, after exposure to a known source of infection, is only about five days. (Vaché.)

This interval is only to be explained by the supposition that germs, of some kind, have gained a footing on shore, and have germinated and grown more numerous. *It is the crop in the hold which produces the first set of cases. It is the crop on the land which causes the second.*

It is only through the action of some organic cause, that we can explain the tenacity of the attachment of yellow fever to certain ships, and these, too, among the cleanest and best aired vessels in the British service. The Sybille had three several epidemic attacks between the 23d of June, 1829, and the middle of April, 1830. Two of these occurred while at sea. In the West India service, certain ships have usually an outbreak on going into even a healthy harbor.

Perhaps no disease has so much puzzled the etiologist as cholera. Its singular local origin, its yet more singular progress, its apparent inconsistencies, its diffusion from a tropical point over the habitable globe, and especially its invasion, in winter, of the frozen steppes of Tartary and Russia, all tend to confuse the observer of epidemics. At one time, slowly, against the monsoon, it advances on a long geographical line, at the rate of from one to two miles a day, whilst at another, it flies on the wings of commerce, almost as fast as there are means of conveyance for men and merchandize. At one time, it ascends or descends along the valley of an innavigable stream, slowly and regularly, as if progressive by its own locomotion; at another, it flies with the ship or the locomotive, across seas and continents. A stranded vessel throws it upon the shore of a lonely sea-island, (Dickson.) One ship conveys it from Dublin to the St. Lawrence,* another meets it *in the midst of the Atlantic,* and carries it to New York,† while a third, from the same source,‡ deposits it at New Orleans. Steamers scatter it far and wide as they ascend from New Orleans to the various branches of the river above. Contagion might explain the progress, where there are always materials to form a line of march, but contagion cannot account for its solitary advance over untravelled wastes or untenanted seas. Contagion cannot explain its presence in the atmosphere of the mid-ocean, nor its manner of assailing a city at once, at its most opposite points. Contagion is at fault as explanatory of the *exemption of classes,* the almost exclusive invasion of low, damp, dirty habitations, and the uniform appearance of a general premonitory state, before the irruption of the cholera itself.

The attacks of cholera within a few hours after exposure to infection, the introduction into hospitals of large

---

* The Carricks.   † The packet ship New York.

‡ The ship Swanton, Captain Duncan, from the healthy port of Havre, was assailed by cholera after being at sea for twenty-eight days, (Lat. 25° N., Long. 57° W.,) and after losing fifteen persons in thirteen days, she arrived in the Mississippi, five days before the epidemic outbreak at New Orleans.

The Ship New York, also from Havre, was attacked at sea, sixteen days out, and arrived at Staten Island, two days before the cholera appeared at the New York Quarantine Station. (Whiting.)

numbers of cholera-patients, whilst the old inmates enjoyed complete immunity, as at the Odinka, at St. Petersburgh, the diseased condition of a single vessel, the Dreadnaught, in the Thames, in 1837, the great exemption of physicians and nurses, the attack of the old rather than of the young, or of those at puberty, all militate against the notion of a propagation by contagion.

On the other hand, many cases are cited where the cholera came with bodies of men, caravans, and ships, and seemed to be propagated by personal communication. At one time it confined itself to one wing of an army; at another, it spread progressively from left to right, along the line of encampment. Sometimes it affected but one out of thirty men in each of a great number of large tents, and sometimes it restricted itself to one or two such tents, which it completely desolated. No wonder that men were puzzled and perplexed, being contagionists at one time and place, and anti-contagionists at another. No wonder that Mojon and Holland should have endeavored to avoid the difficulty by reverting to the exploded doctrine of Kircher and Linnæus, the animalcular theory of disease.

The animalcular, being an organic theory, would explain well enough, the phenomena of progress, were it not for the apparent absurdity of supposing that animalculæ of tropical origin could exist and procreate in a Russian winter. The want of proof that animalculæ are poisonous, or that they fulfil the conditions for such a theory, has been already stated.

But if we assume for cholera a fungous origin, all difficulties vanish; and, as in the case of yellow fever, an easy explanation may be given of every apparent incongruity. We have only to suppose, what is known to hap-

10

pen in other cases, that the fungi, on which cholera is
assumed to depend, acquire at times, as do the germs of
some contagious diseases, an unusual power of reproduction and diffusion, a greater potency of expansion. Such
germs may be carried by men, and goods, and ships, or
may make a slower progress by their own unaided activity, or be scattered by the winds, to regerminate,
wherever special conditions are found. Thus can we see
why the poison prefers the route of streams, or infests
the damp parts of cities; and why classes living in clean
apartments in dry districts, suffer so little.

We can see why women escape better than men, why
both cholera and yellow fever, by the natural tendency of
the vegetable cause to the organs of generation, almost always cause miscarriage of pregnant women, and why,
when a city or country is unhealthy, the fungiferous
causes of death, by over-stimulating the organs of reproduction, usually make a compensation by the births, for
the unusual mortality.

Can we not thus explain the appearance of contagion,
where there is no contagion, and the absence of contagion
while there is an obvious conveyance of the epidemic poison from place to place?

We are no longer surprised to learn that cholera advanced regularly from the tent nearest to the water, to
the others successively, until it reached the end of the
lines; nor do we feel astonished that it was, in another
case, confined to the tent nearest the tank, or to the flank
company, or the brigade on the left or right of the army.
We now see why ninety men detached from a large corps,
and attacked on the first night of absence, on the borders
of a lake, were, without damage to the corps, promiscu-
ously mingled again with it, after being brought back,

totally disabled, to the original encampment. We can understand now, how, in the Odinka Hospital, whose salubrity was previously proved by the absence of cholera during an epidemic at St. Petersburgh, its eight hundred inmates continued in their usual health, despite the introduction from without of five hundred cases of cholera. We can see how a corps, in its march through an irregularly infected country, may acquire and lose the cholera several times; how a healthy corps may enter a sickly army, *en route*, and not suffer from the prevailing malady. The diffusion, the limitation, the leaving the infection behind, or the carrying it forward, all admit of an easy explanation, if we assume the hypothesis that germs or spores, created exteriorly to the body, are the *seminia morbi*, and that they are liable to the usual accidents by which seeds are conveyed, or lost, or favored or repressed.

It would now weary you, my young friends, were I to carry you over the same twice-trodden ground, in an endeavor to apply to the phenomena of the origination and propagation of THE PLAGUE, the same explanatory theory. It fits it quite as well, nay, in some respects even more perfectly than it does the etiology of cholera and yellow fever, but, after what has been said, you can yourselves make the application.

In pursuit of our task of explanation, I am bound to give a reason for the extraordinary exemption of Brazil, New Holland, and the Polynesian Islands, from malarious diseases. They are volcanic, or organic, or alluvial. They have rank vegetation, and heat and moisture, as demanded by McCulloch, and sulphur-products as called for by Daniel and Gardiner, and a soil in process of drying after being wet, as suggested by Ferguson. They have the exuberance of vegeto-organic life of Armstrong and Doughty, and yet they are not infested by malarious diseases. Not a shadow of explanation, do any of these hypotheses offer of this anomaly. But if we assume the fungous theory as a basis of explanation, we may readily believe, nay, *certainly might know*, that such exceptions are, on the doctrine of chances, to be expected. No plant is everywhere, and such plants as are here alluded to, are especially capricious in habits and actions, according to causes which, though yet unstudied, obviously control them. On our theory, *the occasional exception should be looked for;* on any general chemical, or mechanical, or atmospheric theory, *it is inexplicable.* Under such a view, we are not astonished at finding Brazil healthy and Africa pestilential; for their obvious, much more their minute vegetation, is so dissimilar as to render a difference in their invisible phytology highly probable.

These considerations naturally lead us to inquire why the febrile diseases of various countries differ so much. Why have we no yellow fever in Brazil, or India, or Egypt, and why no plague in Florida or Calcutta? It is for the reason, that, though of the same great general class, the fungi differ greatly from each other in special properties, and that the protophytes of each country, although many of them are nearly alike, present some of them, almost contrasted properties. The *agaricus clypeatus* of the west of Europe, poisons in one way, the *amanita muscaria* of Siberia in another. One irritates, the other intoxicates. So, a certain kind of *mucor* produces dysentery, another typhoid symptoms, and a third excessive vomiting. The ergot of rye excites formication, fever and sphacelation, the ergot of maize, fever, loss of hair and nails. Is it then, a matter of special wonder, if a fungus with one set of properties, should germinate in India, another in Egypt, and a third in Cuba.

Nor should we be astonished at finding a surprising fecundity at certain times in certain classes of plants, by means of which they not only multiply prodigiously on their customary soil, but readily advance beyond their wonted boundaries. In this way I may explain the ravages of the plague in Europe, and of the yellow fever in North America and Spain; and account for the intrusion of cholera upon European ground, and its failure to maintain its conquests for any prolonged period of time. The plague retreats back to the Nile, Euphrates,* and Danube, its native home, the cholera withdraws to Hindostan, and the yellow fever to the southern coast of America and to the West Indies. It is twenty-six years since yellow fever visited Philadelphia. During that time, there have been many seasons of as great heat and drought as in 1793 and 1798, and, every year, arrive at our wharves, vessels from infected ports; but the germs of disease do not bear transportation always, and our fungiferous tendencies at home have not invited a visit. Long may it so be in both respects!

To speak of quarantine regulations, does not come properly within the scope of my subject, but the importance of the question may perhaps excuse me for the suggestion that, on the principles here laid down, the detention at quarantine even of the sick, is, for yellow fever and cholera, unnecessary; while the importance of detaining

* At Erzeroum, the capital of Armenia, the winters are cold, the thermometer rarely rising above 32° F. and descending often as low as 25° or even 20°. In summer the heat has a range of from 66° to 81° 5—; yet this place and its adjacent villages, seem to generate the plague. It appeared there in 1840, about the middle of August, and in 1841, in the beginning of July.

10*

and purifying cargoes and soiled baggage, becomes apparently more imperative.

I alluded, in the last paragraph, to the fungiferous tendencies at home, by which, may be invited from abroad,
an exotic *fungus.* This idea affords an explanation of a
fact universally noticed, but not easily otherwise explained.
I mean the growth of various diseases of a common character, before the irruption of a great pestilence. If these
depend upon a fungous origin, their growth will be augmented by the augmentation of their cause, until the
foreign intruder, urged by a new and inherent impulse,
and welcomed by a domestic facilitation, enters upon a
career of desolation. The fungiferous exaltation is
shown by the early ripening and imperfect maturation of
fruits and even roots, whose organs of reproduction are,
by invisible ergots, over-stimulated. The decay of roots
and fruits, the tainting of meats, and the moulding of
other things, are but parts of the unwholesome "cryptogamism," which at length, intrudes upon living things;
when murrain among cattle, and pestilence among men,
complete the history of a calamitous period.

Similar principles seem to govern the movements of
diseases now generally acknowledged to proceed from
germs. The contagious maladies, small-pox, measles,
scarlatina and hooping-cough, are almost always present
in some part of a great metropolis, or at least in some
part of a great country; yet their tendency to propagation
is often, for years, so slight as to confine their ravages to
a small number of victims. But at times, and sometimes
after long intervals of comparative inactivity, these affections suddenly acquire a wondrous expansibility. Their
germs are scattered far and wide. The slightest exposure
brings on disease, and where but a few individuals suffered,

thousands are attacked. A careful examination of the meteorological conditions affords no shadow of explanation. At all temperatures, in every variety of humidity, beneath every kind of skyey influence, these diseases become epidemic. Time seems to have for them some kind of bonds, for they seldom continue epidemic long, and do not usually return as such, for a lapse of years. According to Humboldt, small-pox becomes epidemic in South America, about once in from fifteen to twenty years, and that sometimes without a known re-introduction. These outbreaks seem to depend rather on germinal power than extrinsic enforcement, and remind one of the locusts, which, though every year present in small numbers, appear by myriads at periods of from seven to seventeen years. As the larvæ of these insects lie deeply buried in the earth, beyond the reach of anything but the mean annual moisture and temperature, which are but slightly varied, we have yet to learn what spell it is, which calls them in countless throngs, into active existence.

The plague-spell has not darkened the portals of Christian Europe for more than one hundred years, and the *sudor anglicanus* has not floated on its fetid mists, since the House of Tudor resigned to the Stuarts the throne of England. But these genii of a former age are but asleep. Their time is not yet. When they shall again recover their germinal vigor, and pass beyond their wonted limits, or awake from their long repose, they will retain probably, as before, their new activity or more extended dominion, for a series of years. It is true that a happier age, in comfort and cleanliness, and medical knowledge, has arrived to check their progress, and to limit their deadliness; but it is vain to hope that any disease has been entirely eradicated, or any germ totally lost. In a few

years the cholera will, according to pestilential usage, re-
tire to its old limits, and there perhaps seem to expire,
until forgotten and contemned, it will, after a long repose,
burst again over the fields of India, and the realms of
Europe and America.*

* Since this paragraph was written the cholera *has* returned to Europe
and America, unchanged in character, and unmodified in severity Again,
it haunts damp rural places, and offensive urban localities. Again, it selects its victims from amongst the poor, who are destitute of the oppor-
tunity of defending themselves from the circumambiency of the provoca-
tives of infection. Filth, dampness, and innutrition ; fatigue, bad habits,
and neglect of premonitions, doom these unfortunates to the superadded
evils of pestilence, torture, and death.

LECTURE VI.

EXPLANATORY CHARACTER OF OUR THEORY—CONTRAST OF THE HEALTH OF SEASONS AND PLACES.—SUDDEN ONSETS IN AFRICA.—THE MAREMMA—VOLCANIC ERUPTIONS.—SPUR TO VEGETATION.—REVOLUTIONS IN LOCAL HEALTH.—FAIRY RINGS.—NON-RECURRENCE OF SOME DISEASES.—LIEBIG'S THEORY.—EPIDEMIC MOST FATAL AT ITS ONSET.—DRY SANDY PLAINS SICKLY.—RECAPITULATION.

INDEPENDENTLY of any observable cause, the crops of various kinds differ in a remarkable manner in different seasons. Most of you must have seen the wonderful production of the fruits of all kinds in certain autumns. A year or two since, the trees actually bent down and broke under the immense load of apples, which were left to rot in the fields in many places, for want of the means of securing them. No cause for this exuberance was observable. Farmers sometimes have good crops even in opposition to the inclemency of the season, and as often, under the most auspicious meteorology, are chagrined at the unaccountable shriveling, or paucity of their grain. So is it with the fungi, which, in opposition to hostile meteoration, spring up in unusual places, or abound prodigiously in customary positions. Thus in 1798, a year of protracted heat and drought, Condie and Folwell reported, as remarkable, the abundant production of various classes of mushrooms.

So, were there unaccountable moulds and mildews, in the driest periods of the pestilential years, in New York, Philadelphia, and Natchez. Sometimes but one kind of germ is stimulated, as in the case of the apples already cited, sometimes many are excited, as in some years of great and general "pomonal" luxuriancy. So is it with the fungi, as manifested by the extension of only one disease, or the co-existence of many. Of all plants, the cryptogami are the most capricious, or most susceptible of modification by unseen causes. Hence the quality of the season is scarcely ever an index to the morbid condition of any particular year, although heat, moisture and a redundant vegetation are general precursors of malarious action.

We can, on our hypothesis, easily explain the arrival of the annual morbid orgasm, *after* the rains of one country, and *in* the rains of another. Whether hot or cool, wet or dry, the sickly season is the harvest time of the fungi, which lie tied by time and not by circumstance, until their customary period of activity has arrived; when more or less stimulated by moisture, and food, and electricity, they show a feeble or a strong fecundity.

On our supposition alone, can we account for the sudden effect, in Africa, of the first rains. The dry season bakes the earth to a crust. The lesser vegetation is dried up under the scorching glare of a tropical sun, and nature seems almost at a stand. That is there, the season of health. But the rains commence, and almost in a moment, arises a morbid influence inexplicable by reference either to heat or moisture, or any ordinary decomposition. "The rain had scarcely commenced," says Mungo Park, "before many of the soldiers were affected with vomiting. Others fell asleep, and seemed *as if intoxicated*. I felt a strong inclination to sleep during the storm, and as soon as it was over, I fell asleep on the wet ground, although I used every exertion to keep myself awake. Twelve of the soldiers were ill *next day.*" Only some of the fungi, whose rapidity of growth is wonderful, and whose power of causing vomiting, drowsiness and intoxication is acknowledged, can be plausibly brought to explain the phenomena described by Park. The very sudden production of excessive mould on everything, so as to rot to its centre in forty-eight hours, a piece of cloth or leather, evinced the fungiferous force of the African rainy season. Moisture and heat alone could not produce such effects, for in Brazil no such phenomena are observed or recorded, although the rains are as heavy and the temperature even a little higher.

Contrasted with Africa, is a spot almost as unhealthy as "The Coast." While the latter is low, wet, marshy and filled with the rankest vegetation, the Maremma of Tuscany and the Roman States is high, dry, free from perceptible moisture, and used chiefly as pasture-grounds, which are in no respect unusually fertile or productive. Yet the Maremma, throughout its extended domain of nearly one hundred miles in length, is scourged by the most intense forms of malarious fevers. The campagna di Roma, so celebrated for its pernicious fevers, is included in the Maremma.

This apparent deviation from the healthfulness, which should pertain to a country so dry, and so free from marshes and streams, has always presented to the miasmatists an especial stumbling block ; and a clever writer seems to think that a general malarious theory cannot be accredited by the profession, which will not explain satisfactorily the cause of the unexpected insalubrity of the Maremma.

The surface of the Maremma is formed throughout of

volcanic tufa, which, when sufficiently softened, forms a pasturage, on which feed large herds of cattle. It contains the finest pastures of Italy, on the soil of which are commingled the ordure of cattle and the disintegrated tufa. The former is known to be a favorite growing ground of the fungi, and the latter, I shall now proceed to show, is even better calculated for the same offices.

According to M. Roques, the fine mushroom, *polyporus tuberaster*, of the Italians, grows in the environs of Naples, upon a species of volcanic tufa, very porous and of an argillo-calcareous nature. In the pores of this stone, is deposited the *matrix* of the plant, from which, when moistened and shaded, grow up vast mushrooms, four or five inches high, and eight or ten inches broad. These stones are sent to France and England, where they are used as in Italy, for the production of mushrooms. The English Philosopher, Boyle, first described this stone, under the title of *Lapis Lyncurias ;* "which," to use his own language, "rubbed, moistened, and warmed, will, in a very short time, produce mushrooms fit to be eaten." Old John Hill, who wrote, a century ago, a volume on Materia Medica, published a book entitled "*Lapis Fungifer,*" in which he describes a stone of this kind, in the possession of Lady Stafford. It was a hard, heavy mass, of an irregular shape, and granulated texture, like shagreen leather. This formed the *nidus* for the perennial root of a fungus superior to common mushrooms. One of these fungi weighed, according to Hill, two pounds two ounces, and measured six and a-half inches on the head. The Doctor presumes that the *Lapis Violaceus* of the Germans is of a similar nature.

The Neapolitans bring the tufa used in their horticultural processes, from Calabria, where are found the samples of that volcanic earth, of the finest quality. It is placed for cryptogamous purposes, in shaded excavations, or in natural caves, or in cellars, where, by its means, are produced vast quantities of the best mushrooms.

In the Maremma, where the volcanic tufa is the basis of the soil, the surface is intermixed with the animal remains of departed empires, and the ordure of cattle, is covered with grasses of old pasturages, and is wet with heavy dews. Everything, therefore, conspires there to a fungiferous end. The tufa is fungiferous, the manure is fungiferous, old pastures are always fungiferous, and the dews of the Maremma not only make night fungiferously hideous; but, by their chilly humectation, act as excitants of the train of nervous symptoms, and, as does driving the cattle in the milk-sickness, they bring on an attack, which, but for this element of the *suite*, might have been escaped. Instead, therefore, of being surprised at the ascendancy of malarious diseases in the Maremma, we should feel at a loss for a mode of explaining any want there, of a miasmatic predominancy.

The fungiferous productiveness of the volcanic soil of Italy, is shown by reference to the report of Professor Sanguinetti, Official Inspector of the Fungi at Rome. Not having access to the original, I quote from Dr. Badham's beautiful work on "The Esculent Funguses of England." "For forty days *in autumn*, and for about half that period *every spring*, large quantities of funguses, picked in the immediate vicinity of Rome, from Frascati, Rocca di Papa, and Albano, are brought in at the different gates.

"The return of taxed mushrooms in the city of Rome, gives a yearly average of between 60 and 80,000 pounds weight, and if we double this amount, as we may safely do, in order to include the smaller untaxed parcels, the

11

commercial value is upwards of 2000*l*. sterling. (10,000 dollars.) But the fresh funguses form only a small part of the whole consumption, to which must be added the dried, the pickled, and the preserved."

Thus about 140,000 pounds of mushrooms are *sold* in Rome, a weight equal to that of 175 oxen.

A reference to the fungiferous power of the tufas enables us to explain a hitherto most puzzling fact, as recorded by many authors, and as specifically treated by writers on epidemics. It is remarked by Webster, and Hecker, as well as by other writers, that volcanic eruptions and earthquakes, when productive of disease, do not cause it immediately, nor even in the current year, but usually in that which follows it. If mephitic vapors or gases were the cause of the epidemics in such cases, immediate consequences should ensue; but if the volcanic ashes, or the sulphur and calcareous products, excite the disease by evoking excessively the common cryptogamic growths, or exciting into action, the long slumbering spores of new or unusual protophytes, we ought to find their record in the morbid history of the succeeding year or years. So we learn that the year 79 of our era, was marked *by no unusual mortality*, although Vesuvius darkened, by its ejected ashes, the sun itself, and scattered its products through the atmosphere even to Syria and Africa. Herculaneum and Pompeii were so deeply buried as to be lost for nearly 1700 years, and the soil of Italy, from the Alps to Sicily, was dusted with the furnace-formed products of the volcano. But in the following year, when the now acknowledged fungiferous properties of the tufous ashes could exert on the soil their stimulating influence, disease desolated Italy, and a plague raged with resistless power. That fatal epidemic destroyed daily, for a prolonged season, 10,000 inhabitants of Rome. (Webster.)

One other difficulty remains to be removed, and I shall then, gentlemen, leave this subject for your future consideration, and, if worthy of it, your future investigation. Writers on malaria not unfrequently complain of the unaccountable irregularity of miasmatic action. Attributing, as they usually do, the diseases of the autumn to vegetable or other decomposition, they are disturbed by finding not the slightest relation between the supposed cause and the alleged effect. Heat, moisture, and vegetation being the concurrent elements of their theory, some proportion should be observed between the amount of these, and the intensity or diffusiveness of malaria. But, alas for the speculation, disease sometimes most abounds in seasons remarkable for the negation of the alleged causes. Cool years are healthy, cool years are sickly. Dry years are salubrious, dry years are lethal.* Wet years present the extremes of health and sickness, and years of a mixed character have been in the *plus* and *minus* of the scale of salubrity. Only one element seems to make any approach to a constant relation to the state of health, and that is, *a tendency to excess of vegetable life*. In the autumn of fertile years, there is often the greatest mortality.

Can this arise from the decomposition of the vegetation of that year, which has just been completed? Does the vegetation submit, in the open air, to so rapid a change as that which is to be admitted, to rationally entertain the malarious theory, as usually received? I think not, and farther, the occurrence of severe malarious diseases in barren places, on rocky heights, and sandy plains, shows that we may more rationally attribute the diseases of

---

* "For at Newtown, Long Island, and in most parts of this island, these diseases have existed in seasons of the greatest drought." (Hosack.)

fertile seasons, rather to the spur given to the general vegetation, which is also communicated to the *cryptogamia*, than to a decomposition, which remains without proof, and which, when obviously most active, fails to excite disease.

As the fungi grow at the end of the phenogamous season, their production depends on causes which may or may not have been felt by the common vegetation. Hence, disease seems in this aspect, of inscrutable origination, unless we look exclusively to the causes which may excite vegetation throughout a season, or only in the spring and summer, or only in the autumn.

There is a kind of corollary to the last proposition. Places of malarious character often become, at least for a time, quite salubrious, and places which have, for a long course of time, been healthy, unexpectedly and without apparent alterations, acquire morbid conditions. The streams run at their mean height, the pools are filled to their common capacity, the vegetation seems to follow its wonted course; but the health varies according to unseen influences, for all visible and measureable events move in a customary round. These diversities of salubrity are unexplained by the geology, the agriculture, the climate and the meteorology, which, remaining the same, or moving in defined and customary cycles of obvious similitude, leave no evidence of having any effect on the morbid irregularities. It would seem as if the unknown cause were migratory, or had long fits of irregular repose. Now, we *know* of nothing which possesses an acknowledged power of creating febrile diseases, by which such irregularity can be explained, save by reference to the habits of the fungi.

The cryptogami have, in a high degree, the curious property of destroying their own reproductive powers, or of poisoning against themselves the soil in which they grow. The *lapis fungifer* or volcanic tufa, if actively employed, loses, in about three or four years, its power of production, which is only reacquired by a repose of several seasons. To this peculiarity is now ascribed the production of what are, in Europe, called *Fairy Rings.* These curious denuded circles, amidst the vivid green of an English common, were once attributed to the tiny feet of fairies, who were supposed to make the spots, so marked, their place of revelry. Subsequently they were thought to be the effect of electrical action. Now they are known to be produced by the eccentric growth of various kinds of fungi, and might, therefore, be properly termed the vegetable ringworms of the fields; or rather the ring-plants of the commons. Commencing, as do the ringworms, at a spot, these fungi move progressively outwards, leaving a bare unvegetating space behind them, upon which neither fungi nor grass will grow for a time. Finally, the grass returns, and filling up the centre, follows the protophytes, so as to produce a broad circular belt of scorched earth, which grows more and more in diameter. The fungi, evolved only on the outer edge of the belt, do not again attack the centre, in which the soil appears to have lost its power of sustaining them.

Most persons attribute this fact to the probable exhaustion from the soil of some special element necessary to the growth of these fungi. That this view is erroneous, may be inferred from the observed decay of the fungi on the spot where they grow, by which the elements of their composition are restored to the soil at once.* Besides, if such elements were removed and not thus restored, it is not easy

* The ploughing in of crops of clover is one of the best expedients for the enrichment of the soil. Land is impoverished only by removing its products.

to see, how that soil could ever regain them by repose. But if we suppose the deposit of poisonous *exuviæ* in the soil, by these plants, we can understand how time, reactions, and soaking rains, may remove them, and again permit a reproduction, where, for a time, it is prevented. A curious exemplification of the poisoning of the soil against their own growth is afforded by the fungi which have so lately preyed on the potato-crop. In Ireland the potatoes grow much better in the subsequent year, when the diseased potatoes have been left to rot in the soil, than when they are carefully removed.

We have other analogies for this idea. Macaire, who has given much scientific attention to the effect of plants upon soils, observes, that certain vegetables enrich the earth by their *exuviæ*, as, for example, the leguminous vegetables excrete much mucilage, and thus fertilize it for the *gramineæ*, but that the *papaveraceæ* injure the soil by the deposit of opiate-like substances, and thus prevent or render growths imperfect. So is it with the peach and bitter-almond trees, which, as well as other plants, that produce prussic acid and the poisonous hydrocyanates, render the soil in which they grow incapable of successive crops of the same kind of trees. A nursery in which young peach trees have been planted, and from which they have been soon removed, will not sustain the same kind of stock for eight or ten years afterwards.* Nature thus secures a variety, by a succession of dissimilar vegetations. I might multiply examples; but these are enough for our present purpose. In this way are the fairy rings formed, and in this way are the grasses protected from the end-

---

* Manuring the soil from which a peach tree has been removed, does not mend the matter; removal of the soil, or long repose, will alone suffice.

less destructive ravages of their enemies, as is the human body from the recurrence of violent diseases.

This view may explain the gradual extinction, or unexpected reappearance of trees, shrubs and flowers. The Prim, a New England hedge-bush, began to fail, according to Webster, in 1775, and finally perished. In 1664, commenced the mildew in wheat, in New England, which long rendered it impossible to cultivate that grain on the Atlantic coast of three Eastern States. So have the Morillo cherry tree, the Buttonwood tree, the Linden, and some others, begun to decay, some in one way, some in another. The peach tree is unhappily dying off in New Jersey, so that, perhaps, in a few years, we may have to look exclusively to the South for that delicious fruit.

Of all the known vegetable productions, the fungi appear to have the greatest variety of abating and destroying conditions. They poison their own soil, they depend for luxuriancy on nice contingencies, they are the food of many insects, who eat them up spores and stems, whilst they prey voraciously on one another, fungus being superimposed on fungus, in an almost indefinite series.

Thus, then, may we not improbably account for the occasional disappearance and reproduction of malarious diseases in malarious situations.

The obstruction to their own reproduction on the part of fungous vegetables may be, I speak it with great hesitation, the cause of the non-recurrence of certain violent diseases, such as yellow fever; while it may analogically explain the non-recurrence of diseases produced by contagious germs, such as small-pox, measles, &c.

May I be pardoned here for a short digression? Liebig has attempted to elucidate this difficult point by a chemical explanation. He avers that each contagious disease is produced by the action of a species of ferment peculiar to it, upon as peculiar a matter contained in the solids or the fluids of the body; by which means said matter is consumed, and thus, is a reproduction of the disease prevented by the want of the material upon which the morbid action may be founded. This famous theory of the cause of the production and non-recurrence of certain contagious diseases, has great plausibility and a charming simplicity. It is, also, supported by analogies deduced from the fermentation of gluten, in the production of bread, and that of saccharine matter in the generation of alcohol. The fermentable substances having been consumed, the process ceases, and, without the super-addition of new materials, cannot be renewed.

The objections to the theory of Liebig are both numerous and, I think, unanswerable. The existence of the fermentable matters, as well as of the ferment, is purely hypothetical, no proof being offered of the detection of either. It must, also, be observed, that there is, on this hypothesis, a peculiar substance to be acted on, for each of many diseases. Thus there must be one for *variola*, one for *rubeola*, one for *varicella*, one for *scarlatina*, one for *pertussis*, one for yellow fever, and one for every other non-recurrent disorder. Each of these substances must reside in the system without necessity, and apparently without cause. No influence seems to be exerted by them on the health or structure before disease comes, and their elimination leaves the system unaffected subsequently. But there is presented to my mind a still more important objection, which may be thus stated. For example, every one knows that persons who take small-pox in the natural way, have, usually, severe attacks, a multitude of pustules, and, according to the theory, a very extensive fermentation, and a reproduction of a large quantity of the products of the fermentation. Of course, there has been consumed a great mass of the peculiar fermentable substance, on the pre-existence of which, the susceptibility to small-pox was founded. In inoculated cases, as a general rule, the disease is milder, the pustules are much less numerous, and the peculiar matter is consumed in much smaller quantity, while the products are consequently less. A vaccination produces, usually, only one small vesicle. Its fermenting power consumes, therefore, but a minute amount of matter, and produces but little *virus*. Yet, commonly, by each of these processes, the peculiar fermentable material is *totally consumed*, and the person is commonly protected from a subsequent attack of small-pox.

This objection to the theory of a ferment, seems unanswerable. But it may be strengthened by adverting to the fact, that by making many insertions of vaccine virus in different parts of the body, we may act on a great deal of the fermentable matter, or, by making but one or a few, we may consume but little. Yet, in either case, no one pretends to say that the degree of protection, or the liability to a re-vaccination is altered. These objections, while they unsettle the hypothetical basis of Liebig's explanation, totally destroy its theoretical conclusions. A peculiar matter is assumed as existing, is supposed to be consumed, and not to be usually reproducible. This matter, however, may be equally well consumed by a small or great fermentation, its own quantity seeming to have no relation to the extent or activity of the process, which is governed solely by the mode of using the ferment. How will the analogy, upon which the whole theory rests, sustain the argument of the great chemist? There is a certain quantity of gluten to be consumed in pannification, the action upon it of a ferment, by which the whole is changed, must be ever the same in amount, although it may not require exactly the same time. If the process be less active, it must be proportionally prolonged; if it be more energetic, it will be completed in a shorter time. But the more violent action of a *variola* is not sooner at an end than the gentler process of a *vaccinia*, both requiring for their completeness about the same period of time.

Taking it now for granted, that the chemical theory will not satisfy the physiologist or pathologist, I will proceed to make an argument for the non-recurrence, as producible by the leaving in the system the *exuviæ* of germs. A reference to former parts of these lectures show, that many plants, and especially protophytes, poison, against themselves, the soil in which they grow; and that thus we may, not unsatisfactorily, explain the apparent capriciousness, as to health, of both places and seasons. Supposing that the cell-germs, animal as well as vegetable, possess a like power when they grow in the animal frame, we can plausibly account for several things not otherwise explicable at all. Thus we may presume that some of these *exuviæ* having no emunctory capable of their elimination, remain always where the diseased processes left them; and thus stand as an obstacle to the future action of similar germs.* We can thus, and thus only, say why certain contagious diseases cannot recur, and why certain diseases which are not contagious, as yellow fever, for example, possess a like disability. Their germs having once reacted in the body leave behind a poison, or, at least, an

---

* Syphilitic poison lurks unexpressed in the system for years, or through life, exemplifying itself only in the offspring. So gout leaps over a generation, in which, however, its cause must be ever present, though latent.

impediment, by which their future reaction is there prevented.

But certain contagious, and even non-contagious diseases, obviously dependent on germs, have the power of recurrence for many times. Yet even these are subject, at least temporarily, to the same law; for, otherwise, none of these diseases could have a termination. The impedimental matter being either emulged or decomposed, after a period, shorter or longer, according to each disease, leaves the system open to a reinfection; and thus *syphilis*, *favus*, and *aphthæ* may, for many successive times, disturb the health of the same individual.

Returning to the immediate object of the present lecture, I proceed to explain why it is that the first cases of an epidemic are usually so much more fatal than those which follow them. This is especially true of the diseases of a miasmatic character and non-contagious maladies, such as yellow fever and cholera. Toxication, when of vegetable origin, is made less potent by habit. Thus, in process of time the habitual drinker or opium eater, tolerates enormous doses of alcohol or opium. Nay, even when made as obviously drunk even to insensibility, the old toper is in less immediate danger than the beginner. His organism recovers better, and while the novice dies poisoned or apoplectic, the snoring habitual drunkard recovers from his coma and cerebral congestion. Thus is it with those who are toxicated by an atmospherically conveyed fungous poison. At first it proves eminently fatal; subsequently, although its symptomatic expression may be as strong, its danger steadily decreases, until at length almost every case recovers.

For this reason, medical men, at the commencement of a violent epidemic, are driven too often from a treatment founded on proper principles, into a loose and dangerous empiricism. For the same reason, are they disposed, at a later period of the attack, to rely upon means of cure obviously inert, or improper, because, the lessened mortality smiles an approval. Let any one found his treatment from the first, upon a proper knowledge of the pathology, and a decent regard to prominent symptoms, and he will succeed in the end, not only much better, but also much more satisfactorily to himself, than those who lower themselves to the level of mere empirics. The deaths are at first owing, not to the greater potency of the cause, but to the keener susceptibility of the recipient of disease. While it increases the severity of the cases, this susceptibility is not greater for our remedies, and therefore we must necessarily have, at the outset, less success.

The malarious diseases commonly found in the rich alluvial courses of rivers, or shores of lakes, sometimes abound on sandy plains. Several writers describe the sickly plains of Brabant as superficially dry and almost bare of vegetation, and Dr. Ferguson informs us of the desolate aspect of Rosenthal and Oosterhout, in South Holland, where a level sandy plain bore nothing save some stunted heath-plants. Beneath the surface, was found at no great depth clear potable water. The plain on the side of the river opposite to Lisbon, dreaded for its pestilential character, is also dry and sandy. Here no ordinary vegetation, no decomposition, can explain to us the cause of this malign power. But there is a teeming vegetation beneath, and almost at, the surface of such places, to which alone can we attribute their diseases. Truffles, a species of mushrooms, grow prodigiously in such places. They delight in sandy plains, and their microscopic congeners are also there in abundance. Such plains, in our own southern country, emit a fungous or mouldy odor,* soon after night; which fact has not a little puzzled curious observers.

May not the healthful power of the plough be mainly attributed to its destruction of fungous growths of this, and of other kinds. Almost every writer on malaria, speaks of the beneficial influence upon health, of a constant cultivation. Now, we know, that when a country is covered with woods, it is usually salubrious, and that when cleared, and put under imperfect tillage, it becomes more sickly; but that a regular system of husbandry by the plough, restores to it all its former healthfulness; while the placing it for some time in pasturage, causes it to again retrograde to a certain degree. The plough is the especial enemy of the fungi, which, either beneath the surface, as truffles, or upon it, as mushrooms, are obviously lessened or extirpated by the constant disturbance of an active tillage. Nothing else known to be capable of affecting the health of the inhabitants, is materially altered by agricultural processes.

I have now, gentlemen, brought to a close the prolonged examination of the cause of miasmatic fevers, and non-contagious epidemics. Let me recapitulate, in a very cursory way, the most important elements of our argument.

I began, by showing that all the usually received opinions on this subject, are liable to insuperable objections, except that which refers to the causation by organic life, and especially by animalcules, as held by Columella, Kircher, Linnæus, Mojon, and Henry Holland.

* This is, probably, the cause of the musky odor noticed by Humboldt, when the soil of some tropical regions is disturbed.

While I was impressed, for the reasons so ably stated by Holland, with the greater probability of the organic theory, I prefer, for reasons stated by myself, the fungous, to the animalcular hypothesis.

My preference is founded on the vast number, extraordinary variety, minuteness, diffusion and climatic peculiarities of the fungi.

The spores of these plants are not only numerous, minute, and indefinitely diffused, but they are so like to animal cells, as to have the power of penetrating into, and germinating upon, the most interior tissues of the human body.

Introduced into the body through the stomach, or by the skin or lungs, cryptogamous poisons were shown to produce diseases of a febrile character, intermittent, remittent and continued; which were most successfully treated by wine and bark.

Many cutaneous diseases, such as *favus* and *mentagra*, are proved to be dependent upon cryptogamous vegetations; and even the disease of the mucous membrane, termed aphthæ, arises from the presence of minute fungi.

As microscopic investigations become more minute, we discover protophytes in diseases, where, until our own time, their existence was not even suspected, as in the discharges of some kinds of dysentery, and in the *sarcina* of pyrosis. We are therefore entitled to believe that discovery will be, on this subject, progressive.

The detection of the origin of the muscardine of the silk worm, and a great many analogous diseases of insects, fishes and reptiles, and the demonstration of the cryptogamism of these maladies, their contagious character in one species of animals, their transfer to many other species, nay even to vegetables themselves, all concur to

render less improbable, the agency of fungi in the causation of diseases of a febrile character.

A curious citation was subsequently made, of the fungiferous condition during epidemics and epizootics. These
moulds, red, white, yellow, gray, or even black, stained
garments, utensils and pavements, made the fogs fetid,
and caused disagreeable odors and spots, even in the recesses of closets and the interior of trunks and desks.

These moulds existed, even when the hygrometric state
did not give to the air any unusual moisture for their sus-
tentation and propagation. Their germs seemed to have,
as have epidemics, an inherent power of extension.

The singular prevalence of malarious diseases in the
autumn, is best explained by supposing them to be produced by the fungi, which grow most commonly at the
same season. The season of greatest photophytic activity,
is, in every country, the period of the greatest malarious
disturbance. The sickly season is, in the rains in Africa,
in the very dry season in Majorca and Sardinia, in the
rainy season of the insular West Indies, and in the dry
season of Demerara and Surinam. Even when the vegetation is peculiarly controlled, as in Egypt by the Nile,
and the cryptogami are thus thrown into the season of
winter and spring, that season becomes, contrary to rule,
the pestilential part of the year.

Marshes are a safe residence by day, whilst they are
often highly dangerous by night. In the most deadly
localities of our southern country, and of Africa, the
sportsman may tread the mazes of a swamp safely by day,
although at every step, he extricates vast quantities of the
gases, which lie entangled in mud and vegetable mould.
This point, so readily explained by reference to the acknowledged nocturnal growth and power of the fungi, is
a complete stumbling-block to the miasmatists.

The cryptogamous theory well explains the obstruction to the progress of malaria offered by a road, a wall, a screen of trees, a veil or a gauze curtain.

It also accounts for the nice localization of an ague, or yellow fever, or cholera, and the want of power in steady winds to convey malarious diseases into the heart of a city, from the adjacent country.

It explains also well, the security afforded by artificially drying the air of malarious places, the exemption of cooks and smiths from the sweating sickness, the cause of the danger from mouldy sheets, and of the sternutation from old books and papers.

On no other theory can we so well account, if account at all, for the phenomena of milzbrand and milk-sickness, the introduction of yellow fever into northern ports, and the wonderful irregularities of the progress of cholera.

The cryptogamous theory will well explain the peculiar domestication of different diseases in different regions, which have a similar climate; the plague of Egypt, the yellow fever of the Antilles, and the cholera of India. It accounts, too, for their occasional expansion into unaccustomed places, and their retreat back to their original haunts.

Our hypothesis will also enable us to tell, why malarious sickness is disproportionate to the character of the seasons; why it infests some tropical countries and spares others; why the dry Maremma abounds with fevers, while the wet shores of Brazil and Australia actually luxuriate in healthfulness. The prolonged incubative period, the frequent relapses of intermittents, and the latency of the malarious poisons for months, can only be well explained by adopting the theory of a fungous causation.

Finally, it explains the cause of the non-recurrence of

very potent maladies, better than the chemical theory of
Liebig; and shows why the earliest cases of an epidemic
are commonly the most fatal.

When I entered upon the task of elucidating for you
this very difficult subject, gentlemen, I did not dream of
its extent and importance, nor did I suppose that it would
have imposed upon me so much research, or inflicted upon
you so many lectures.

I have, therefore, not attempted to account by this theory, for the periodicity of malarious diseases, rather for
want of time than want of power, and from a desire not
to tax too severely your patience.

The task is now completed. Yet, after all my labor
and your polite attention, the theory presented to you, may
not be finally demonstrated. But it is the most consistent
with the phenomena known at present, and is much better
sustained by established facts than any other hypothesis
yet presented to the world. It has, therefore, the requisites
of a philosophical theory, which, in other and more exact
sciences, would be accepted, not to be held as absolutely
true, but as, in the present state of our knowledge, the
most plausible and convenient explanation of the phenomena.

It has another value. It will revive the inquiry into
the causes of fever, by giving to it a new direction, by
offering new points of view, new motives for study and
new lights from analogy. If, too, its confirmation or re-
futation should give to future inquirers after truth, half
the pleasure which I have derived from excursions into
this new field of mingled reason and fancy, these Lectures
will not have been vainly elaborated.

THE END.

MEMOIR
ON THE NATURE
OF MIASM AND CONTAGION

John L. Riddell

Art. V. — Memoir on the nature of Miasm and Contagion.

Read to the Cincinnati Medical Society, Feb. 3d, 1836. By
John L. Riddell, Adjunct Professor of Chemistry, and
Lecturer on Botany in the Cincinnati Medical College.

The age in which we live is distinguished over all that have
preceded it, in the advances that have been made in the
physical sciences. Men seem to have become convinced,
that little value can attach to abstract generalizations; and
that the true mode of studying nature, is by following

patiently in her footsteps, watching her silent progress, and developing her manifold and harmonious ways by experimental inquiry. Nature is limitless; — man is finite: — consequently there must be boundless fields of ever-during truth, unmarked by the footsteps of man, and unseen by the telescopic vision of research. Even within what we call the circle of human knowledge, blanks are met with, wide and dreary, and regions which seem shrouded in perennial mist. In contemplating the phenomena of nature, the mind is ever prone to fill up these vacuities with creations of its own; and then combining the real with the imaginary, the known with the unknown, to mould the whole into the form of a general system. But the experience of the world has clearly shown, that hypotheses embracing wide ranges of facts or principles, are exceedingly liable to prove more or less erroneous. They should, therefore, in all cases, be held liable to amendments, to modifications, or even to entire dismissal, upon the development of new facts making such requisitions.

Proudly as we boast of the investigating spirit of the times, very many of the theories and opinions which at this day obtain general assent, had their origin in the dark ages of science, and have been borne down to us by the current of tradition. New and relevant truths are from time to time brought to light, indicating in some instances the propriety of their total abandonment; but the fascinated minds of men are wedded to the prevalent hypotheses, and but too often, the requirements of venerable systems are mistaken for the immutable laws of nature. The novel facts are perhaps doubted, controverted, overlooked, deemed anomalous, or made to bend and accommodate themselves to the favorite theory.

The leading views I am about to offer, have been suggested at various times and by various writers. If I mistake not, however, it has always been unfashionable to believe in them, and still more so to advocate them. When the science of physiology was infinitely more vague than it is now, ere the genius of a Hunter or a Cuvier had brought to light the structure of the lower tribes of beings, or the microscope revealed its atomic worlds of animate wonders; while chemistry was yet in its feeble infancy, before the nature of the atmosphere had been investigated, or the laws of union in definite proportions determined; then might such doctrines have been considered as resting on slender probabilities. But at this time, with the multiplied results of careful observation and skilful experiment before us, it is certainly far otherwise: wherefore in venturing to stem the current of popular opinion, brooking the intolerance of some, and the ridicule of others, I feel upborne by the consciousness, that my conclusions are indicated by analogies the most clear, and facts the most incontrovertible.

I assume that the matter of contagion is of an *organized* nature, and consequently subject to the same general laws, which regulate the origin, increase, modes of existence, and duration of animal or vegetable bodies. I assume also, that the same is true of the morbific miasms which are exhaled from putrid marshes, and of the occult causes of cholera and other epidemic diseases.

In order that due weight may be assigned to the facts and arguments on which this hypothesis rests, I will first notice some of the prominent points of contrast between organized and inorganic bodies. Organized beings, animals and plants, possess forms more or less rounded, and never exceed in size certain definite dimensions:—mineral or inorganic bodies as a class, have no general determinate form, unless it be the angular one assumed by them in the crystalline condition, and in respect to their size, there are seldom any assignable limits. Organized bodies are made up essentially of the ultimate elements, oxygen, hydrogen, and carbon; or of oxygen, hydrogen, carbon, and nitrogen; in all cases united in a most complicated manner. The composition of individual minerals is always characterized by definiteness and comparative simplicity, though as a class, they embrace all known elementary bodies.

Minerals increase in size by the external addition of particles similar to their own; and the causes which elaborate and supply these particles, are wholly independent of the bodies which they tend to augment. Animals and vegetables possess within themselves a power of elaboration; they consequently increase in size by the internal assimilation of foreign particles. In all organic structures of the more highly developed types, there exist harmonious and dependent series of vessels, tissues, and organs, which concur in effecting this end. Of this internal conformation, minerals are wholly devoid. The same causes which develope and perfect the organic structure, ultimately put a limit to the duration of individual beings;—whereas all brute matter is endued with the negative attributes and conditions requisite to insure endless perpetuity. Though a finite period of existence is allotted to individual plants and animals, it is believed by many that nature has fixed no bounds to the duration of species. Cuvier and Roget recognize this opinion as a settled point in physiology;—yet I confess it is more consonant with what seems to me the general ways of nature, to suppose that particular species or kinds lose their identity in process of time, by giving origin to modified kinds or varieties; which in turn may long wear the aspect of confirmed species, and ultimately, in like manner, give way to their successors. However this may be, there is certainly no assignable limit to the reproduction, succession, and continuation of organized beings.

I claim for the corpuscles which cause malarious and infectious maladies, trans-microscopic as they are, the humble rank of belonging near the lower confines of organic nature. Perhaps they hold nearly the same grade in respect to animate and sentient beings, which the more simple and minute of the *Fungi* and *Algæ* do to the more perfect tribes of vegetables. Inconceivably minute as they doubtless are, they must yet possess a share of vitality, because like other animals and plants which come under our observation, they have the power of propagating and extending themselves indefinitely. With a view of throwing light by analogy on the possible habitudes of miasmatic molecules, and demonstrating at the same time the strange and almost incredible capabilities of animal life, I shall adduce a few well authenticated observations on the nature and habits of infusory animalcules:— though in honesty I do not imagine there exist very close resemblances between the animalcules which the microscope displays to our view, and the miasmatic corpuscles which elude its cognizance.

Infusoria is the name of an obscure class of the animal kingdom, characterized more by the minuteness of the beings it embraces, than by any particular features or structure which they possess in common. This appellation was proposed by the Danish naturalist, Muller, distinguished for his acquaintance with this department of zoology, on account of the fact, that myriads of these little creatures always make their appearance in fermenting infusions of animal or vegetable matter. They are, by no means, however, confined to such infusions, being frequently met with on the leaden tiles of houses, in putrefying sores and depraved humors of man and beast, and in one, at least, of the healthy animal fluids. Countless multitudes of a parti-colored, eel-like animalcule, (*Vibrio tritici,*) exist in the pulverulent substance within the glumes of blighted wheat. Dr. Lindley, of the University of London, says, (First Principle of Botany, 329,) that the granules of pollen, (the fecundating dust, elaborated by the flowers of plants,) inclose a mucuous substance, in which is contained an infinite number of exceedingly minute molecular bodies, having a power of active motion. It is now generally believed, that animalcules do not occur in pure fountain water, nor in many of the healthy animal fluids. To account for the occurrence of these animated atoms in particular situations, baffles the most untiring ingenuity of research. Spallanzani made some instructive experiments with a view of determining the condition preclusive of, as well as those most favorable to their production. He placed portions of the same vegetable infusion in different glass vessels. Some were left exposed to the air, others slightly covered, and others hermetically sealed. He found, subsequently, the

3

greatest numbers of infusoria, in those vessels which were most freely exposed, yet they occurred in the infusions hermetically sealed. Boiling the infusion, though it reduced their numbers, did not entirely prevent their appearing. In one instance he boiled the infusion for an hour, and then hermetically sealed it: after the lapse of twenty-five days, a a few of the smaller kinds of animalcules had been developed. They readily appear under reduced pressure, where the air will support only thirteen inches of mercury.

Some species of animalcules have the power of enduring great changes of temperature in the medium containing them, with apparent impunity. The *Vermiculi tauri*, which inhabit a medium of 103 deg. Fahr., support 5 deg. without death, and retain their vivacity a long time at 32 deg., the freezing point of water. The same beings are not destroyed by raising the temperature to 133 deg. The native medium of the *Vermiculi hominis*, is usually maintained at 98 deg. These vermiculi retain vitality between 32 and 131 deg. The common infusory animalcules are capable of brooking a range of temperature, from the freezing of water, to near 110 deg.

Collateral facts, drawn from the vegetable kingdom, show, in a manner equally striking, the great power sometimes possessed by organic nature, of enduring extremes of heat or cold. Immense fields of scarlet snow, are sometimes presented to the traveller, in the intensely cold regions of the northern frigid zone. Investigation has shown, that the color depends upon millions of microscopic plants, belonging to the order *Fungi*. The *Ulva thermalis*, a plant of the order *Algæ*, and the *Limneus pereger*, a fresh water shell, are found in Gastein thermal springs, where the constant temperature is 117 deg. (De la Beche, p. 18.)

The most mysterious circumstance in the natural history of the infusoria, is the susceptibility which some of them possess, of remaining an indefinitely long time in a perfectly dry, and seemingly lifeless condition.

The same prerogative is enjoyed, to a certain extent, by many vegetable seeds, and by certain worms of the order

Annelida; but the resurrection of animalcules, taking place more rapidly, is far more striking to the observer. " The *Rotifer redivivus,* or wheel animalcule, which was first observed by Lewenhoeck, and was afterwards rendered celebrated by the experiments made upon it by Spallanzani, can live only in water, and is commonly found in that which has remained stagnant for some time in the gutters of houses. But it may be deprived of this fluid, and reduced to perfect dryness, so that all the functions of life may be completely suspended, yet without the destruction of the vital principle; for this atom of dust, after remaining for years in a dry state, may be revived in a few minutes by being supplied with water. This alternate suspension and restoration of life may be repeated, without apparent injury to the animalcule, for a great number of times. Similar phenomena are presented by the *Vibrio tritici,* an eel-like animalcule, which infests diseased wheat, and which, when dried, appears in the form of a fine powder. On being moistened it soon resumes its living and active state.

The *Gordius aquaticus,* or hair worm, which inhabits stagnant pools, and which remains in a dry and apparently lifeless state when the pond is evaporated, will, in like manner, revive in a very short time, on being again immersed in water. The same phenomenon is exhibited by the *Filaria,* a thread-like parasitic worm, infesting the cornea of the horse." (Roget. Physiology. I. 58.)

In the Edinburgh Encyclopedia, article Animalcule, it is stated, that the wheel animalcules have been thus resuscitated from a state of dormant vitality, as many as seventeen times in succession, and that the presence of sand is necessary in the fluid, or they will not revive. That when active, 113 deg. is sufficient to kill them, but when dry, the vital principle is not destroyed unless the temperature be raised to 158 deg.; or if, while in this condition, they be exposed to the intense cold of — 11 deg., they may be subsequently revived. Strong camphoric and terebinthinate odors prevents reanimation.

In no other department of animated nature, are we pre‐sented with such strange and anomalous modes of reproduc‐tion. Many of the globular *Monades* and *Vorticellæ*, increase by spontaneous and equal division. The living globule will at first appear as if encircled by an equatorial band, which will continue to be drawn more and more tight, until a complete separation occurs; each portion being an independent monad, which in turn is bisected like its parent. In this manner, a mysterious multiplication goes on indefinitely. The *Monas uva* consists of four or five corpuscles in a cluster, by the spontaneous separation of which, the species is propagated. Errhenberg has determined that the smaller monads are near one twenty‐four thousandth of an inch in diameter; and he has estimated that there are 500,000,000 of them in the space of a cubic line, or drop of liquid which he examined.

The *Volvox globator* consists of a spherical, membranous sac, filled with liquid, in which float many more diminutive globules like itself. These have precisely the same structure with the enveloping membrane, even to containing within them a series of still minuter spherules. Observers have thus seen the fifth generation in the same individual. The parent always ends its own existence in giving birth to its progeny. The *Gonium pectorale* has an angular, flattened body, containing sixteen corpuscles, which subsequently become distinct animalcules like those in the volvox. A curious being, provided with a beak, was observed by M. Bonnet, in an infusion of hemp, which fixing itself to some solid substance, assumes a spherical form, and rotates irregularly until it bursts into four animalcules. Spallanzani took pains to isolate the egg of an animalcule on a watch glass: in a short time it was developed, became mature, and produced eggs like the one from which it sprung; and these likewise followed the same habits.

It is indeed astonishing to observe how short a time is sufficient, in some instances, to bring these beings to full maturity. An infusion of beet yields a species that increases by detaching obliquely a small piece of its own substance, which, after the lapse of a single day, is also capable of propagating. Strange as this may appear, the instance is less remarkable than that of the *Vorticella ramosa,* which exercises the power of reproduction, within a few hours only, after having been itself ushered into existence.

So far as investigation has been carried, this proposition is fairly established: that animal or vegetable food is essential to every subject of the animal kingdom. It must therefore follow, if the proposition be universally true, that the *Infusoria* feed on organic substances; and it is probable, that many of them subsist on corpuscles more minute than themselves. Some of them are known, indeed to be carniverous. To adduce an instance, Goeze has seen the *Trichoda cimex,* a bristly, microscopic creature, of an oval form, seize upon and devour the lesser animalcules with great voraciousness.

A belief in the existence of miasmata, or morbific agents in the atmosphere, has long been entertained. When the general constitution of common air was discovered and announced to the world, it was expected that a prolific source of maladies would be found in the varying proportions of its ingredients; but repeated and careful analyses have demonstrated, that the relative quantities of oygen and nitrogen are found to be nearly constant, whether the air be taken from the infected wards of a crowded hospital, from the most pestilential marsh, or from the most pleasant and healthy situation. True, the quantity of carbonic acid in atmospheric air, varies at times from one per cent. to one in a thousand; but these variations seem to have no connexion with the prevalence or production of disease. The amount of miasmatic matter diffused through infected air, must be almost inappreciably small. M. Boussingault, of Lyon, has lately made a series of most careful experiments on the composition of air, procured from highly malarious districts. He has determined the presence of hydrogen, not existing as a constituent of water, to an extent by weight, varying from three to eight millionths of the air examined. He presumes, from other important experiments, that it was a part of something of an organic nature.

In these instances, portions of air were submitted to trial, which, though they contained less than a hundred thousandth part of any thing that could be called miasm, were nevertheless sufficiently imbued with the germs of disease to give rise to the most severe intermittent fevers. So, likewise, the remote cause of cholera may lurk, unappreciated, in the atmosphere. It is well known, that a quantity of contagion, as the virus of small pox, altogether too minute to affect the most delicate balance, is sufficient to develope a disease in the human system, which may propagate itself to an indefinite extent.

A grand and most decisive argument, relative to the probable nature of infectious miasms, may be drawn from the established laws of chemical action and combination. Multiplied researches have demonstrated, that when elementary or compound bodies chemically combine, it is invariably in certain fixed and definite proportions; thus, 108 parts of silver unite with 8 parts of oxygen; 40 parts of potassium with 8, and also with 16 parts of oxygen; 40 parts of sulphuric acid combine with 48 of potash. Consequently, substances, in producing chemical effects, lose *pari passu* the affection or power which enables them to do it: in the same manner as a moving body parts with its momentum in giving motion to other bodies. Suppose I endure, for a while, the action of a drachm of the concentrated solution of caustic potash, on the palm of my hand. The presence of the alkali will cause the decomposition of the dermoid tissues, the elements of which, will be converted into oleic, margaric, and stearic acids, that immediately combine with, and neutralize the causticity of the potash: and thus, at length, the potash will have a limit put to its action, its place being supplied by the various soap-like salts to which it gives origin, and of whose composition it forms a part.

It is after this wise, that the action of every possible dead substance must have a definite limit. A small quantity of such an agent produces only a comparatively small effect, while a large quantity produces an effect correspondingly large. The unpleasant ulcer which would follow the application of caustic potash to the hand, could not be communicated to other persons by contact;—the morbific cause would not in the slightest degree possess the power of self-propagation.

There is, then, this wide difference between contagious and ordinary poisons, that in the one, the extent of the effect depends wholly upon the quantity of material employed: in the other, the smallest possible quantity is adequate to the production of the greatest possible effect; an effect which may be felt, as in the case of small pox, by millions of human beings. The chemist has power to produce all mineral or inorganic combinations at pleasure, though unable to imitate the more complex results of vital action. Now, if the causes of pestilence be inorganic, why has the virus of small pox, the miasm of cholera, or of any other pestilential malady never chanced to originate in chemical laboratories?

Must there not then, be a degree of vitality resident in the matter of contagion? Is there not a perfect analogy between its unlimited propagation, and the unlimited propagation of animal or vegetable species? What brute force, let me ask, within the compass of inorganic nature, acts unexpended? and where may we find this high prerogative, except as a mysterious endowment of vitality?

The virus of many contagious diseases may be kept in a dry condition for a very long time, being still capable of exciting disease by inoculation. How perfectly similar this is, to the wonderful resurrection of which the dry and shapeless remnants of certain animalcules are capable; and how totally inexplicable on any other hypothesis.

Miasmatic poisons, when applied to the animal system, generally require several days, before the obvious development of any effect. This time, called the latent period, affords a strong argument in favor of the organized nature of the poison; for ordinary poisons never delay their action so long: whereas, if contagion consists of living corpuscles, like the ova of insects or the germs of plants, they would naturally require time for their development and multiplication.

The interesting experiments of Moscati and Boussingault, have shown in my opinion beyond a doubt, that organic matter exists in extremely small quantities, in the noxious air that hovers over marshes.   Moscati, a learned Italian, many years ago, suspended in the air, over the rice grounds of Tuscany, a globular glass vessel, filled with ice.   An abundant deposition of dew took place upon its surface, which, when collected, appeared at first to be pure and limpid water.   There was soon, however, an appearance of little flakes, " possessed of properties peculiar to animalized matters, and, finally, at the end of some days, the liquid putrified completely."

M. Boussingault, in a memoir read to the French academy of Sciences, in August, 1834, details some striking experiments made by him at Cartago, South America.   "A little after sunset," says he, "I placed two watch glasses on a table standing in the middle of a swampy meadow.   In one of the glasses I poured hot distilled water, in order to wet its surface, and, at the same time, to communicate to it a temperature higher than that of the air.   The cold glass, its temperature being lowered by the nocturnal radiation, was soon covered with an abundant dew.   The warm glass could not evidently condense dew.   On adding a drop of distilled sulphuric acid to each glass, and evaporating to dryness with the heat of an alcahol lamp, I always saw a trace of carbonaceous matter adhering to the glass in which the dew had been deposited, while the glass which had not condensed dew, was perfectly clean after the volatilization of the acid."   I may here add, that strong sulphuric acid decomposes and blackens organic matters, in consequence of its affinity for water; causing the oxygen and hydrogen of those substances to unite in the production of water, and leaving the carbon in the condition of finely divided charaoal, which accounts for the occurrence of the black color.   The same writer further says, that he soon experienced upon himself the effects of the miasm, whose presence he was endeavoring to prove: for he was attacked with a fever which forced him to interrupt his researches.

(Concluded under the head of Original Intelligence.)

Art. IV.—Memoir on the nature of Miasm and Contagion.

Read to the Cincinnati Medical Society, Feb. 3*d*, 1836. By
John L. Riddell, Adjunct Professor of Chemistry, and
Lecturer on Botany in the Cincinnati Medical College.

(Concluded from page 412.)

To use his own language, " the results obtained prove very
clearly that, in marshy places, during the precipitation of
dew, there is an organic matter deposited with it."

Since most of this memoir was in type, I have made some
experiments with a view of detecting the aerial miasm of
small pox. A perfectly clean ounce phial was half filled
with distilled water; a small glass tube with a capillary ori-
fice was made to terminate near the bottom, the upper and
much larger portion of the tube bending horizontally to receive the silver nozle of a delicate pair of bellows. Several
turns of gauze were passed around the mouth of the phial
embracing the tube, and the whole was securely fixed in an
appropriate wooden frame-work.

On the fifteenth of February the apparatus was carried to the city pest house, and under the superintendence of Dr. O. M. Herron, it was placed on a table two or three feet from a small pox patient, just in that stage of the disease when the circumambient air is supposed to be most contagious. The bellows were blown by the nurses pretty constantly, for twelve hours, thus presenting a great amount of noxious air to the distilled water. The apparatus was left undisturbed until it came into my hands three days after, when I made the following experiments:

1. One fourth of a drachm of the water contained in the phial, evaporated very slowly in a watch glass, over an alcohol lamp, left concentric circles of a whitish substance. Upon bringing this residue under the object glass of a good microscope, I discovered that it consisted mostly of long crystals, which shot from each other at right angles. The outer margin of each concentric band was less distinctly crystalline, and evidently contained some other substance.

2. A minute drop of sulphuric acid, (carefully distilled and collected on a glass rod, so as not to leave the slightest trace upon being evaporated from clean glass,) was placed upon some of the residue, (experiment No. 1.) Upon the application of heat the acid became black, and upon complete evaporation a dark stain was left; thus showing the presence of organic matter.

3. Upon adding a drop of pure sulphuric acid to near an eighth of a drachm of the water, and expelling the water by a careful heat, the acid became black. This experiment, as well as the one which follows, was performed upon a piece of Florence flask, rinsed in clean water and then heated to redness over an alcohol lamp, in order to remove every trace of organic matter.

4. A drop of the water hastily evaporated, left a whitish residue, not crystalline to appearance, but consisting of extremely minute grains. Upon the application of a high heat short of redness, it became dark colored, indicating the presence of organic matter, by the charcoal liberated. A still

higher heat, in contact with air, removed the dark color and left a mere trace of white adherent powder.

These results compel us to believe, that organic matter was communicated to the distilled water by the air which was transmitted through it. This matter did not exist in the air by virtue of its volatility, else in the first experiment it would have been dissipated by evaporation. It was most likely in the form of organized corpuscles, sustained in the air by their exceeding small size.

I was somewhat puzzled with the appearance of crystals in the first experiment, not expecting to see anything more than a gelatinous substance. Upon examining distilled water subsequently, through which the human breath had been passed for several hours, a tissue of delicate arborescent crystals was left after evaporation. I have only time to offer a crude and premature conjecture. May not these saline matters have been borne mechanically into the air, in the one case, muriate of soda from the perspiration of the patient, in the other, a saline substance exhaled in respiration?

About two drachms of the water through which variolous air had been passed, was hermetically sealed in a clean glass tube, leaving a space filled with air above the liquid, equal to one fifth its capacity. The tube has been kept upright in a situation where the temperature is pretty constantly 72 deg. Fahr. An ash-colored sediment soon appeared, which continues to increase. Examined with the microscope a week after it was first adjusted, the sediment appears to consist of numerous, irregular, partly filamentous, ragged masses, with here and there a perfect globule about twice the size of the globules of human blood. The filaments, which may be seen with the naked eye, are seldom arranged in a regular branching manner. After all, we cannot consider these experiments as decisive; for it is evident that in transmitting air even through a capillary tube, mites and filaments of organic dust from the bed clothes etc., may have been sent into the water and retained.

A great law seems to pervade and control all nature, as we rise above the lifeless aggregate, occult, indeed, and incomprehensible in its cause, but not the less obvious in its effects. I refer to the degeneration of races. One race or variety will flourish and endure for a time; but at length it begins to degenerate, and is finally succeeded by other kindred varieties, which have their day, and in like manner yield their places. From the influence of this grand custom, even man himself is not exempt. The Indian is fast disappearing from the forests and plains of America, and where stood his rude wigwam, or where he made war upon the beasts of the wilderness, the white man builds his house, or taxes the fertile soil for the means of wealth and comfort. The mastodons, plesiosauri, and gigantic cycadeæ, of very ancient times are now unknown upon the earth. They are extinct, and beings of modified structure and different habits have succeeded them. Illustrations of this law are constantly presented for our contemplation, in the limited duration and decline of esteemed varieties of fruits and esculent roots; as in the apple, pear, potatoe and yam.

The temporary predominance of certain insect races, of which there are many striking instances on record, seems to have a relevancy to the present subject. I will merely cite a few facts which came under my personal observation. In the spring of 1833, the leaves of the buckeye (*Æsculus ohioensis*) were infested and devoured to an incredible extent, in Franklin county, Ohio, by the larvæ of a small yellow miller. So far as I know, the buckeye has not been infested since.

Some twelve or fifteen years ago, I well remember, that for a mile or two on each side of the Chenango river, New York, every individual sugar maple (*Acer saccharinum*) was destroyed by the depredation of a large caterpillar, which, neither before nor since, has ever made its appearance in sufficient numbers to attract common observation. No thinking mind, I imagine, will fail to trace a close analogy, between the temporary prevalence and anomalous succession of epidemic diseases, and the occasional appearance, in such vast numbers of these destructive races of insects.

Bearing in mind the modifications of which animal races are susceptible, under the influence of altered circumstances, and recollecting the brief hours and minutes which are sufficient to give full maturity to certain animalcules, we may, perhaps, understand why, when the same epidemics prevail at intervals of many years, they are apt to assume different aspects; being at one time quite mild, at another attended with great mortality; giving origin to symptoms in some instances which are unknown in others.

If, then, we admit the presence of living corpuscles in miasmatic air, there are many who would be inclined to suppose, that these corpuscles must possess a very complex organization, to enable them to maintain themselves in that medium. The presence of external organs equivalent to wings, might, by some, be deemed necessary to effect that end. We have, however, the best of all possible reasons, short of demonstration to the senses, for believing that no such necessity exists:—a reason drawn from mechanical philosophy.

Bodies when of very small dimensions, no matter how dense their texture, encounter a degree of resistance in falling through material media, which essentially retards their velocity. Larger bodies do not experience this resistance in so great a degree, because they present less surface in proportion to their weight. Very minute bodies, in falling through the atmosphere, soon acquire nearly a maximum velocity, which they do not exceed until they reach the earth. Dr. Thompson, in his late work on heat and electricity, says that globules of water, the thousandth part of an inch in diameter, acquire by falling through the air, a maximum velocity of nine or ten feet per second. Recognising the laws which regulate the descent of bodies in resisting media, and presuming the miasmatic corpuscles to have the specific gravity of water, I have made calculations to determine the velocity with which one of the monads, measured by Errhenberg, would be capable of falling, through such a medium as common air. The diameter of these creatures is

$\frac{1}{24000}$ of an inch:—one of them would fall near four feet per second.* A corpuscle $\frac{1}{1440000000}$ of an inch in diameter, would fall one inch per second, or five feet in a minute's time. It is therefore easy to imagine, that wingless beings, of transcendent minuteness, may float securely in the subtle air, or be borne on the wings of the winds to the most remote regions of the earth.

In the winter of 1833, I prepared several bottles of water, from clean, recently fallen snow. They were tightly corked, and kept for three or four months in the shaded corner of a room, where the water was not liable to be frozen. At the expiration of this time, having occasion to use some of the water, I observed that the lower portion of each bottle was traversed by myriads of delicate, dark colored filaments, bearing a close resemblance to some of the fresh water algæ. Upon removing the cork, a most unpleasant odor was exhaled, similar to that of animal putrefaction. No one, I presume will doubt, that the living germs of this curious organization came down from the high regions of the atmosphere, in conjunction with the snow.

The doctrine I have espoused might be elucidated still farther, if need be, by analogies from the vegetable kingdom. Perhaps nearly all the true diseases to which plants are liable, arise from encroachment by parasitic fungi and lichens. The rust which infests the culms of wheat, was found by Sir James E. Smith, to consist of highly organized microscopic fungi. We hardly know a single species of the more perfect plants, on whose mature leaves, may not at times, by careful

---

*In obtaining these results, gravity is regarded as a constant force, and the air as of uniform density. Put $d = \frac{1}{1000}$ of an inch, $v =$ its maximum velocity, 10 feet per second, $m =$ diameter of the monad, $x =$ maximum velocity of the monad per second.

Required, the value of x in terms of d, v, and m.

The falling body acquires its maximum velocity, when resistance $=$ gravity. Resistance is as the square of the diameter and square of the velocity:— gravity is proportioned to the cube of the diameter.

Now, as the elements of resistance $d^2\ v^2$: to the element of gravity $d^3 :: m^2\ x^2 : m^3$. Therefore, $d^2\ v^2\ m^3 = m^2\ x^2\ d^3$. $x^2 = m\ v^2 \div d$. $x = (m\ v^2 \div d)^{\frac{1}{2}} = 4\frac{1}{2}$ feet, when $m = \frac{1}{24000}$ inch.

examination, be discovered some minute and obscure species of this order; and I question much whether a tree can be found in the forest, on whose bark cannot be seen the spreading and parti-colored lichen.

In like manner do parasitic growths affect animal bodies. Do not warts, cancers, sarcomatous tumors, hydatids, and intestinal worms, possess an animal vitality insulated from that of the individual in whose body they occur? For myself, I cannot but regard them as holding about the same relation to the animal system, as the parasitic fungi and lichens do to the more completely organized vegetables.

The majority of medical writers now living, have expressed their belief in the existence of terrene and paludal emanations, which they suppose to be of a gaseous and inorganic nature. No doubt it will be often repeated, that it is unphilosophical to recognise vital corpuscles, as morbific agents, before they have been demonstrated to the sight. "Show us your corpuscles or animalcules, before you call on us to believe in their existence." In reply, it may be said, that we have infinity on either hand; infinite expansion, and infinite minuteness. The range of man's vision, though aided by all the resources of art, is but a point on an infinite line. As well might the skeptic assert, that there were no worlds, no stars, no globes of matter, save what his feeble vision descried; as that the mysterious attributes of life could not attach to beings invisibly small.

A WORD FROM THE PROPRIETORS.

The proprietors design publishing, at the close of the next number, the names of all those who have paid their subscriptions in advance. As the Journal has been irregular in its appearance in the hands of former proprietors, all payments made before the tenth of April shall be appended to the advance list. They are making arrangements for paper made expressly for the work, so that the entire volume will present a uniform appearance, both in letter and paper, as well as improving it in many other respects; consequently, the tenth volume will be attended with additional expense, and hence they hope their subscribers will pay in advance on that vol., at least. Three dollars is but a small sum to one man, while two thousand times that amount is of much importance to those who are daily paying large expenses. The editors and proprietors are determined that their work shall equal any other, both in matter and mechanical execution, in the Union. In future they expect to be responsible for the appearance of the work. Price 4 dollars at the close of the vol.. 3 dollars and 50 cents at the end of three months, or 3 dollars in advance or within the first quarter.

JOHNSON & WOOD.

YELLOW FEVER
CONTRASTED WITH
BILIOUS FEVER

Reasons For Believing It a
Disease Sui Generis
Its Mode of Propagation; Remote Cause;
Probable Insect or Animalcular Origin, &c.

Josiah C[lark] Nott

III.—*Yellow Fever contrasted with Bilious Fever—Reasons for believing it a disease sui generis—Its mode of Propagation—Remote Cause—Probable insect or animalcular origin, &c.* By Josiah C. Nott, M. D., Mobile, Alabama.

In the April number, 1845, of the American Journal I published an essay on the *Pathology* of Yellow Fever as presented to our notice in Mobile. I now propose to give the results of my observations on the peculiar habits, or what may be called the Natural History of this disease, and my reasons for supposing its specific cause to exist in some form of Insect Life. *Malaria,* which, according to the received doctrine of the day, is a gaseous or molecular emanation from the earth's surface, is, in my opinion, wholly inadequate to the explanation of the mode of propagation of this disease, and I am therefore induced to offer a different solution which is strongly supported by the phenomena attending it. The whole doctrine of Malaria is but an hypothesis, and if we can substitute another for it which is better sustained by reason and analogies, and which conflicts with no known law of nature, it is the part of sound philosophy to give it a preference, until a less objectionable one can be found.

There is no novelty in the doctrine of Insect or Animalcular origin of diseases. Many of the older writers, amongst whom are conspicuous Linnæus, Kircher and Nyander, have promulgated such an opinion, and it has been vaguely presented from time to time to the notice of the profession, but it is only since the publication of Ehrenberg's great work on Infusoria (1838) that its bearings can be fully appreciated. The medical periodicals of late years have made occasional allusions to the subject. Dr. Wood, of Philadelphia, Dr. Watson, of London, and others make honorable mention of it, but the most elaborate and ingenious article I have met with is that in Sir Henry Holland's "Medical Notes" "On the Hypothesis of Insect Life as a cause of Disease."

Sir Henry coyly approaches this *mundus invisibilis* as-an " Hypothesis," and it is well that extreme caution should preside over our medical reasoning, and that undue weight should not be given to ingenious speculations ; but when medical science in its onward course arrives at a point where an old "hypothesis" is inadequate and contradicted by established facts, another theory which is less exposed to these objections and well sustained by analogies may perhaps not improperly be dignified by some appellation a little stronger than that of Hypothesis.

As far as *doctrines* are concerned the history of Medicine is little more than a recital of successive delusions, and we have too much reason to know, that it takes almost as much time to uproot a false medical doctrine as a false religion, when it has once seized upon the public mind. From the time of Hippocrates to that of Lancisi the doctrine of Malaria had no existence, but at length the great revelation " *De noxiis palludium effuviis,"* came, and the world marvelled and was converted. After a while, however, this great dogma began to be scrutinized more closely—doubts and difficulties sprang up and gathered strength as time rolled on—and finally some of the infidels, amongst whom is Dr. John Bell, of Philadelphia, (one of the best medical writers of our country,) have been bold enough to deny the very existence of Malaria in any shape, and have contended that Meteorological changes, radiating and absorbing qualities of soils and plants, dews, &c., are sufficient alone to explain the occurrence of those diseases commonly attributed to Malaria.

Though this subject has for many centuries enlisted no small share of talent, learning and industry, yet has little been done towards dispelling the darkness which overshadows the morbific causes of fevers. A crude mass of facts has been collected, but so contradictory do they seem, that no attempt at systematizing them has yet succeeded—facts however are immutable—the contradictions are probably only apparent, and a careful investigation may show that the errors lie not in false facts, but in false hypotheses.

Malaria has been assumed to be a *Unit,* and *Identity* for all the fevers of hot climates follows as a corollary. Intermittents, Remittents, Congestive and Yellow Fevers are all thrown into this Grand Gulf of morbid Poison—*rari nantes in gurgite vasto.* Here arises a very grave question. If this doctrine of *identity* be wrong, it is clear that the whole history of fevers has been vitiated by false assumptions, all the logic based on false premises; and our chance now for arriving at truth is to go back and ascertain what *are* facts and make our deductions *de novo.* A field is here laid open far too wide for the limits of a Journal, and I must therefore confine myself to the illustration of one division. Though I shall be compelled from the nature of the case, by way of illustration, to allude, *en passant,* to other types, I beg it to be borne in mind that *Yellow* Fever is the subject before me. I regard this as a disease *sui generis,* and though I hope to do more, the establishment of this point alone would be a very important step in the Etiology of Fevers.

Macculloch, who may be regarded as the *ipse agmen* of the Malaria party, meets the question fully and fairly in the following proposition: " Whatever Malaria may be in its simple state, it is only as united to the atmosphere that we know it, and we must therefore view it as an æriform fluid, as far as the question of its propagation is concerned. It must be considered as the very atmosphere itself, when it exists ; and *its propagation therefore must be primarily regulated by those laws which govern the motions of currents of air.*" Here one of the important issues is placed upon its true ground, and by this it should be fairly tested.

When then we have exhausted all the known laws which regulate the atmosphere, and which appertain to gases is general—when, too, we have exhausted all the known and supposable habitudes of molecular emanations of vapors and dews, and are still unable to account for the propagation or transmission from point to point of Yellow Fever, the idea of Malaria must so far be abandoned. It is not permitted to *assume* new laws, which are subversive of others that are known.

I propose now to show, from facts presented during the various Epidemics in Mobile, that the morbific cause of Yellow Fever is not amenable to any of the laws of gases, vapors, emanations, &c., but has an inherent power of propagation, independent of the motions of the atmosphere, and which accords in many respects with the peculiar habits and instincts of Insects.

I must here anticipate the main discussion by laying down a few leading facts in relation to the manner in which Yellow Fever *has been* propagated in Mobile on various occasions, as these facts form the groundwork of much which follows, and must be frequently alluded to.

The town of Mobile, which contains about 15,000 inhabitants, is situated at the mouth of the Mobile River where it enters into the Bay. It stands on a plain composed of sand, here and there a little clay, with vegetable matter and shells. The whole formation is evidently alluvial, and from the numerous beds of unfossilized *grathodon* and other shells found in the vicinity, and other geological indications of comparatively recent change of level, there can be no doubt that the whole platform around the town has undergone a movement of upheaval at some epoch not very far removed from ours. These beds of shells are found of various elevations—some as much as 20 feet above the river, and are composed of shells which belong to species *now found in our waters*, in a perfect state of preservation. The soil in and around the town is very porous, the water from the heaviest rains disappearing in a few hours. The tides here do not rise more than from one to two feet, and ebb and flow but once in the 24 hours. There is a marsh on the north and another on the south which touch the suburbs. On the west the land gradually rises some 40 or 50 feet for five miles, when it breaks off abruptly into high pine lands.

Though in previous years, when the town was comparatively small, Epidemics were not uncommon, it is a remarkable fact that no Yellow Fever occurred for eight years previous to 1837, except sporadically. Since my removal to the city, (May, 1836,) there has been no year without sporadic cases, and not less than five Epidemics of greater or less magnitude have prevailed, viz: in 1837—'39—'42—'43—'44. I shall select, from the history of each, a few facts bearing on the points to be examined.

The first Epidemic I witnessed was that of 1837, which was announced by a single case on the 10th of September. Four more cases occurred about the 20th, and it is remarkable that all these cases occurred at points so remote from the shipping and so distant from each other as to preclude the idea of recent importation, or propagation by contagion. They seemed to arise, each from an independent focus. The next cases did not appear until about the 10th of October, or some twenty days after the last mentioned cases, when it commenced spreading rapidly in all directions as an Epidemic, and carried off about 350 persons before it was arrested by a "killing frost." There was nothing in the character of the weather to account for the slow progress during the first thirty days, and it assumed the Epidemic character a few days after a very heavy southern gale which caused the water of the river to overflow the low parts of the town on its margin.

The next Epidemic occurred in 1839, and commenced during the first days of August, where it should have been the least expected, viz: on the corner of Government and Hamilton streets, half a mile from the shipping, in a clean, well ventilated and fashionable part of the town. For a short time the disease spread slowly around this focus, but at length it burst forth in every direction with extraordinary violence, ravaging not only the town, but the environs for several miles. This was one of those great Epidemics, in which the disease, shaking off complications, assumes its true and undisguised character, and usurping the field, swallows up every thing else in the shape of Fever. Number of deaths 480. Almost all the seaports on the Gulf were visited by Yellow Fever this season in severe form. There was nothing peculiar in the weather, but on the contrary it had been pleasant, temperate and showery. There was no imaginable cause why the dormant germ of Yellow Fever should have been aroused to such extraordinary activity at so many distant points at the same time.

In 1842 we again see the disease, commencing the 29th of August, in Spanish Alley, a very filthy place near the docks, where it would naturally be expected. From this point it spread with surprising deliberation in a north westerly direction—travelling slowly from house to house, and taking more than a month to reach and extend along Dauphin street, which runs the whole length of the town, dividing it into two equal parts. Its course and progress could be traced step by step, and its ravages were confined to one half of the town, leaving the other almost untouched. Had frost kept off a few weeks longer, there is every reason to believe it would have continued its course and marched over the other half of the town. Another Epidemic appeared in 1843, commencing about the 19th of August in the opposite or northern extreme of the town, and pursuing a course the reverse of the preceding year, viz: south east—taking about the same length of time to extend itself over the northern, that it had over the southern half in 1842—leaving the southern part almost untouched. Number of deaths 240, and checked by a severe frost.

Such was the *general course* of the disease in the last two years, though there were some trivial irregularities. In each of these years persons by visiting the infected district contracted Yellow Fever and carried it home with them to other parts of the city, still the disease was not in any instance communicated or propagated by them. It travelled day by day for weeks, progressing from point to point like the army worm through the cotton region.

In 1844 Yellow Fever made its last appearance in Mobile (except sporadic cases,) but to so limited an extent as scarcely to deserve the name of Epidemic; still the facts are curious and important in connection with our subject. The first cases occurred about the 1st of August, and others continued to appear at irregular intervals for about two months, which were scattered here and there over the town in a very extraordinary manner. The number of deaths was but 40, and they could not have been more scattered, occurring on different squares with apparently as little connexion as would the same number of labor cases.

A review of the Epidemics just detailed, will reveal some curious and important *habits* of Yellow Fever, which have been strangely overlooked by writers on the subject; and so far from being peculiar to that disease in Mobile, its history in other places will show that they belong to it every where. The progress of the disease, in Philadelphia and New York particularly, has been marked by the same peculiarities. I beg leave to call attention especially to the Epidemics of 1842–3, as the mode of propagation in these years forms the basis of all my reasoning. In these years the disease started from a single focus at different extremes of the town, and after hanging about the point of origin for a short time, took up its march and progressed steadily and slowly for more than a month, until it overspread one half of the town, without being stopped by variations of weather.

How is this slow progress to be accounted for? Why did the disease, while the sea and the land breezes were sweeping the town daily in every direction, take a *month* to extend half a mile and then stop in the heart of the town? If the morbific cause exists in the form of *Malaria*, which "*we* only know as united to the atmosphere"—if it can be influenced by currents of air, or propagated by contagion, its course and conduct could not have been such as described. It was literally and truly a *migrating disease*, possessing an inherent power of reproduction and progression irreconcilable with any known laws of gases, emanations, vapors or dews. Even Liebig's theory of *fermentation*, which is the *latest fashion*, is equally insufficient, for a *fermenting* point of the air cannot stand still. Macculloch has discoursed largely about the fantastic motions of the atmosphere; he tells us of upward currents and downward currents—straight, curvilinear and irregular currents—the curious distributions of dews, &c., &c., but all falls short of the mark, however applicable such explanations *may be* to the propagation of *Intermittent* Fevers. Yellow Fever, in 1842 and '43, travelled from house to house for more than a month, as would a tax collector, and was just about as much influenced by the weather; for neither the fever nor the tax collector like to travel in rain, though they pay no regard to the direction of winds.

On the other hand, in the years 1837—'39 and '44, the disease started in succession from several or many foci, and diffusing itself gradually or rapidly in the different years, seemed to lose all connection with the points of departure or origin; cases occurred here and there in every direction. These facts may at first glance seem to contradict those before given; but a little reflection will satisfy the reader that they are all perfectly reconcilable by the Insect theory, and no other.

Before entering on the "Insect Hypothesis" in detail, it may be well to give a familiar illustration of it, based on facts well known to all classes in the cotton region. The perfect analogy between the habits of certain insects and Yellow Fever will thus be made apparent at once.

It is a law of nature that every plant affords sustenance to several parasitic insects, and the average number of each plant has been estimated at half a dozen. The cotton plant like others is attacked by *its* parasites, having their peculiar habits and instincts. One or several of these insects may appear the same season, and true to their instincts each attacks different parts or *organs* of the plant—as the leaves, bark, woody fibre, roots, pods or bolls, flowers, &c. Some years there may be an entire exemption from one of these insects, or to use a medical phrase, there may be a few *sporadic cases.* At another time a worm may appear at a single point, and from this focus will spread slowly over a portion of a field (as did the Yellow Fever in 1842 and '43) leaving the other portion almost untouched. In another year a worm comes like a great Epidemic, appearing at many points in rapid succession or simultaneously, and ravaging not only a single plantation but laying waste the cotton region for several hundred miles. Some of the insects appear on the hill-tops, others in the low places. Some attack the vigorous *plethoric* plants, others the delicate and feeble plants, &c. One planter, a very sensible, accurate observer, informed me that some very minute insect attacked his cotton field last summer in *concentric circles,* causing a very singular appearance; the alternate circles of healthy and diseased plants varying in elevation and resembling the waves of the ocean.

The history of the great *Army Worm* which destroyed the cotton crop of the last year is very curious and instructive. From the best information I can procure, this worm appeared in 1820, in 1840 and 1847, long and irregular intervals. A writer in the July No. of the New Orleans "Commercial Review" has, I think, demonstrated some instructive facts connected with its Natural History. He shows that there is no provision for its preservation during the winters of our climate, and that it must perish so soon as its food, which is the cotton plant alone, is exhausted. He states, also, that this worm commences in the extreme south, and progresses invariably in a north westerly direction. This worm belongs, like the silk worm, to the *Moth Tribe,* and there is a strong similarity in the habits of the two Insects. There is no natural provision *here* for the hybernation of *the* silk worm; it is a native of the tropical climate, and its generations follow each other in rapid succession. It feeds exclusively upon the Mulberry tree, and if the eggs were not preserved by artificial means they would all inevitably perish. When the warm weather of the spring comes on, the eggs require to be kept in a cool, dark place, to prevent them from hatching before their food is ready for them, viz: the leaf of the Mulberry. If the worm is born before the leaf puts forth, it perishes. The case of the *Army Worm* is perfectly analogous—from its known peculiarities it *must be a native of a tropical climate,* where the cotton plant is *perennial.* The time required from birth to full maturity, including all metamorphoses, is but ten days. We have numerous instances of the emigration of butterflies and other insects across water to a great distance, and it is very easy to conceive how the moth, which produces the army worm, might (breeding with the rapidity it does) find its way from Mexico or South America into the southern part of the United States and gradually overrun our cotton region. If, as the writer alluded to, asserts, the time of existence of the Army Worm is but ten days, and its food be exclusively the cotton plant, the conclusion is inevitable that it must come into existence and die in the spring long before their food is produced in our climate.

I have been a little minute in these details, as I shall have occasion to allude to them afterwards when speaking of the migrations and other habits of Yellow Fever and some kindred diseases.

Even this little sketch is sufficient to show some striking analogies between the habits of insects and those of certain Epidemic diseases. Some insects lie dormant for years, and then appear in several or innumerable points, and varying in number from a few up to countless myriads; others appear, but very variable in extent every year. The reasons for their long repose, their irregular and sudden resurrection, their varying numbers, the habitation and condition of their germs, during these different periods, are inexplicable difficulties which remind us strongly of the vagaries of Yellow Fever. The different insects, too, (like Epidemic diseases,) attack different *organs* of plants—at one time very circumscribed in their operations, attacking one or a few spots; and at another, bursting forth like a wide-spread Epidemic. There are no appreciable meteorological changes which can account for "each change of many-colored life."

Animal and vegetable decomposition are governed by laws which are more uniform, more palpable and easily comprehended—whenever animal or vegetable matter is subjected to the action of heat, air and moisture, decomposition rapidly ensues; and there is no summer in our climate during which a dead horse or a bale of hay will not rot in the open air and in a few days throw off plentifully its offensive effluvia. These effluvia too must abound *every* year, (though fevers are but *occasional*) and as Macculloch remarks they become incorporated with the atmosphere, and unlike the *materies morbi* of Yellow Fever, are compelled to obey its motions.

Though my argument is intended particularly to illustrate Yellow Fever, which I regard as a disease *sui generis*, still I may be permitted to remark that the present state of facts do not warrant us in assuming Identity for all the other forms of what are termed Marsh Fevers, viz. Intermittent, Remittent, Bilious and Congestive Fevers. The various and strongly contrasted types described in the United States—those of Flanders, of the different countries lying on the Mediterranean, and those of Africa and India, all of which have been described. may well excite serious doubts on this point. I am by no means sure that all these types may not be most rationally explained by attributing them to various insect species, but laying aside this hypothesis and assuming the *malarial*, it would be a strange anomaly in nature, should it be proven that but one morbific cause of fever is generated over the broad surface of our variously compounded globe.—Fever should have its *genus* and its *species*, like other things in nature.

Though chemistry has arrived at a wonderful perfection in analyzing and separating into their primitive elements the various mineral, vegetable and animal substances which surround us, yet the laboratory has not succeeded in bringing to light any gas or product of putrefaction which can produce in the human frame a train of symptoms resembling those of Periodic or Yellow Fever. Many of the products of the laboratory will disturb health or produce death, but they create symptoms of their own. There are many known facts which make it probable that a *multiplicity* of Malarial poisons exist. It is ascertained that different soils eliminate different gases, as Azote, Sulphuretted Hydrogen, Hydrochloric acid, Hydrogen, Carburetted Hydrogen, Car.

bonic acid gas &c., and yet we have no evidence that any of these have any agency in producing *Fevers.**

Again we have a vast number of *Emanations,* which are known to exist, though beyond the reach of the chemist—for example the various forms of animal matter ; as flesh, fish &c.—the infinite variety of plants, as well as soils, all give off peculiar emanations which are only detected by the sense of smell. There are also other emanations of which we should be wholly ignorant were it not for their effects on the human system. Some of these are mineral, some vegetable and others animal—such as those from Mercury, Lead, Arsenic &c.—those from the Mancinella tree, the Rhus Toxicodendron, the Upas &c.—those from the bodies of persons laboring under contagious diseases &c. &c., and there can be no question that the chapter on Emanations might be greatly extended could we trace all diseases to their causes. But we may well doubt from their *peculiar mode of propagation,* whether the *materies morbi* of " Marsh Fevers " exists in this form.

M. Chervin, in one of his last works " *De l'identité de nature des Fièvres d'origine paludéenne de différents types &c.*" has given the fullest and most labored argument I have met with in favor of the *Identity* of Yellow and Marsh Fevers; and as it is indispensible to my argument that Yellow Fever should be as far as possible isolated, I will introduce his *resumé* as a text for what I have to say on this point. These conclusions will be found at the close of his essay under the caption :   " *Analogies entre les Fièvres Périodiques et la Fièvre Jaune.*"

1st. " Yellow Fever has never prevailed epidemically out of the Tropics except in summer or autumn, that is to say, in those seasons in which Intermittent and Remittent Fevers prevail."—Chervin.

This proposition may be admitted without hesitation, as it proves nothing, if true.

2nd. " Yellow Fever is never seen except in localities where Periodic Fevers may be developed."

If true, this proposition should deserve no more weight in settling the point in dispute, than the last.   The fact that two diseases are always found in the same climates and localities no more proves *identity* for them, than similar circumstances would prove identity for two plants or two animals.   But we have good authority for disputing the *fact* laid down. Yellow Fever *does* occur in localities where Intermittents are extremely rare or *wholly unknown.* Amongst other examples we may cite the Island of Barbadoes, which is thoroughly drained—almost every

---

* Important discoveries might be suggested by the phenomena which occur in sweetening a cup of tea as well as by the fall of an apple.   When a lump of sugar is dropped into a cup of tea numerous bubbles of air, which had occupied its pores, are seen to rise to the surface ; and in riding in the suburbs of Mobile a few weeks ago after very heavy rains I perceived large quantities of gas gurgling through the newly formed small ponds, which was displaced from the porous soil in the same way that the air was from the sugar.   This gas is easily collected after heavy rains, and it would be a curious subject of inquiry to ascertain its composition in different soils and localities.

foot of it in a high state of cultivation and is according to the authorities *exempt* from Intermittent Fevers. Intermittents once prevailed here extensively, but have been exterminated by drainage and cultivation. The fact is notorious that invalids suffering from Periodic Fevers go from the surrounding Islands to Barbadoes to get cured of these disseases, and yet *Yellow* Fever prevails nowhere with more malignity than in Barbadoes.

3rd. When in the Equinoxial regions the Yellow Fever sweeps off the unacclimated population, Periodic Fevers prevail generally amongst the Creoles and old residents."

This opinion has often been advanced and although there is apparently some foundation for it, I think a false interpretation has been given to the facts on which it reposes. Periodic fevers do certainly often occur, to a very *limited extent* in those localities where Yellow fever is seen, and in the same season, but, as before stated, this proves nothing as to their identity. The *unacclimated* population of Mobile, for example, may be simultaneously attacked by the two diseases, whilst the *acclimated* residents, (who are exempt from Yellow fever,) may, if its morbific cause is present, be attacked by Periodic fever, against which there *can be no acclimation.* The extent however to which Intermittents prevail amongst the creoles during Yellow fever Epidemics has been greatly exaggerated by M. Chervin. In Barbadoes these Periodic fevers do not accompany Yellow fever *at all*, and in Charleston, Mobile, and New Orleans they are rare except in the outskirts bordering on the marshes. The physicians of these cities must all sustain me in the assertion that the creoles and other acclimated residents are healthy during Yellow fever Epidemics. Periodic fevers certainly do not "*sévissent généralement contre les créoles et les anciéns residens.*"

4th. " The meteorological phenomena, which exercise so marked an influence over the march of Yellow fever, exert an analogous influence over that of Periodic fevers."

The physicians of our Southern Seaports are certainly not prepared to receive this proposition as demonstrated, for according to our observations the *origin* of Yellow fever at different epochs is entirely independent of appreciable meteorological changes, though after it has once *started* it progresses more rapidly in dry than very wet weather. No one can pretend to predict the occurrence of Yellow fever the day before the first case appears. In Mobile we are often taken by surprise as is the case at the time I am writing (30th July, '47)—a case occurred in a Capt. Smith at the Mansion House, about the 18th of this month, though the weather has been remarkably temperate and the rains have been falling in torrents for a month—cases have occurred in New Orleans in June, under similar circumstances, and in both cities the disease is a month in advance of its usual time of appearance. The disease does not with any regularity therefore appear in the *hot years* as has been asserted, but just as often in the showery pleasant seasons; cases have been occurring every day or two in New Orleans, for the last 6 weeks in the midst of the unceasing rains, but the disease will not probably extend rapidly until the rains cease—if the cause is animalcular we can well imagine how rains may impede their march. But when this disease once gets under way it is unimpeded by winds or storms, and nothing short of a "killing frost" can arrest it—repeated light frosts may come, but the disease continues till arrested by the *freezing point*. If Yellow fever were caused by emanations from decomposing animal or vegetable matter, a single freezing night might *suspend* the elimination of these effluvia ; but the influence must cease when the cause is withdrawn. We often have two or three weeks of weather after a killing frost, as warm as that which preceded it, and there is no reason why the decomposition should not resume its operations ; but not so with the Yellow fever—like in insect life, when the ova are once hatched, the propagation of this disease goes on till arrested by a *killing frost*—and it can only be animated by another summer's sun, which calls from their slumbering places the various insect tribes.

5th. We know that the miasms which give birth to Periodic fevers may be transported by the winds ; so is it with those which produce Yellow fever ; *only in the latter case their deleterious action does not extend so far."*

Even M. Chervin, then, is here forced to admit a distinction between these diseases—viz : that Yellow is *less influenced* by winds than Periodic fevers. But here a question surrounded by fearful difficulties opposes our progress—to what extent are these different diseases influenced by winds ? The writers on *Malaria* present us a strange confusion of facts on this point and time does not permit us to enter as fully into its elucidation as we could wish. It seems to be a generally admitted fact that the morbific cause of Intermittent fever may be wafted several miles, *over land*, whether the *materies morbi* exists in a gaseous or animalcular form ; but when we come to the propagation of Malaria *across water* we become lost in a most extraordinary labyrinth of contradictions !

Macculloch who has written the most elaborate and complete treatise in our language on Malaria, makes no allusion to the commonly received opinion of *absorption of malaria by water ;* and not only gives well authenticated instances where it has been wafted to vessels 5 or 6 miles out at sea, but even goes so far as to attribute the spring Intermittents on the West coast of Great Britain, during the prevalence of Easterly winds, to Malaria which has been borne *across the sea from Holland.* He says that clouds, fogs, swarms of insects, the perfume of cinnamon groves and we might add clouds of dust may be transported by winds long distances ; and if so, why may not the *materies morbi* of Intermittent fever ? The doctrine of Malaria supposes a gaseous poison which rises from the earth and mingles with the atmosphere—it is clear therefore, that in the case alluded to, if there be no *local* cause of malaria on the coast of Great Britain, where these intermittents occur, the Malaria must come from Holland, as it cannot emanate from the sea. Thus, Macculloch argues, must stand the case, or the whole doctrine of Malaria be abandoned. These Intermittents come with the East wind and no other ; and it cannot be maintained that an uncontaminated wind, from any point of the compass, can produce a specific disease. The East wind does not produce Intermittents in other parts of Great Britain or in other countries, and the Intermittents alluded to come only with the East wind.

Opposed to these opinions of McCulloch, which are maintained by a preponderance of authorities, we find a great many of equal respectability contending that *Malaria* cannot be propagated, or transported by winds across water, even a very short distance.

Sir John Pringle, Sir Gilbert Blane, Dr. Fergusson and others, give instances where the most pestiferous fevers could not be transported *a few yards* across water. Notorious examples of this kind have twice occurred in the English Fleet at Walcheren, one of which is related by Sir Gilbert Blane, though he gives an instance in another place of Intermittents attacking vessels several miles from land.

As an example I will select, from many, the following remarks of Sir James Johnson on the fever of the famous Walcheren Expedition.

" Nothing could more clearly *prove the limited range of marsh effluvium* than the contrast between the health of the Navy and that of the Army. Although the ships were distributed along the shores of Walcheren and Beveland, from Flushing to Batz, most of them within *a cable's length* of the banks, yet *no sickness occurred* except amongst such parts of the crews as were employed on shore and *remained there during the nights*. Most of the officers of the ships and many of the men were in the habit of making excursions through all parts of the islands by day with complete immunity from fever. The night was here, as in sultry climates, the period of danger." The entire width of the channel between Walcheren and Beveland is about 6000 feet. The history of fevers so abounds in similar facts that it would be needless to multiply them here.

How strongly do the two classes of facts, referred to by Macculloch and Johnson, contradict each other ; how irreconcileable do they seem, and yet if human testimony be worth any thing, each is sustained by such a chain of testimony as to place it beyond question. As before remarked, the difficulty will probably be found to be in a false " hypothesis" and not in false facts. May not these contradictions be more rationally reconciled by *supposing a plurality of morbific causes to exist?* One rising into, and mingling with the atmosphere and obeying its motions, and another propagating itself by different laws ? How else are we to explain the *facts* that Intermittents *are* transported to distant points and elevated to the height of a thousand or more feet ; while Yellow Fever as certainly *creeps along upon or near the surface of the earth?* Yellow Fever is certainly very often, if not always, stopped in its progress by water, but is not impeded by rows of trees, houses, and other barriers, against Intermittents. There are numerous instances recorded of vessels lying near the wharfs of infected towns, or near other vessels, on board of which, Yellow Fever prevailed violently, without being contaminated. There are even perfectly authenticated instances where *one side or end* of a ship has suffered severely from this disease, whilst the other was entirely free from it ! We can readily believe, that certain insects which are endowed with unaccountable instincts and habits, might attack a part of a ship, of a tree, of a wheat or cotton field ; but we cannot imagine how a gas could be turned loose on one side of the cabin of a vessel and not extend to the other ! ! ! Some new law of gases or emanations must be discovered by the Malaria party before they can explain this mystery.

It would appear that *Malaria* embarrasses its friends very much, not only by the irregularities of its journeyings over water, but by those over dry land. Dr. Robert Williams, the distinguished author of the work on " Morbid Poisons," says, " *different soils* also act as attracting or repelling causes which affect the transmission of the paludal poison." In addition to other similar facts, he tells us that Dr. Morton mentions the following instance in the neighborhood of Weymoth. The inhabitants of a dry district, immediately around, or on a level with the marsh, being nearly exempted from the fever which greatly prevails on the more distant hills. This same fact is also observed on the hills of Sussex." Dr. Williams adds instances of similar import which we might easily multiply. He gives no evidence of this *attraction* of Malaria by the plain, and if he were at all *practically* familiar with paludal Fevers in hot climates, he could not have advanced such an idea; for it is a well known fact in our Southern States that the morbific cause of Intermittent or Remittent Fevers will almost invariably pass *over the* low lands, *no matter what may be the character of the soil*, to attack the neighboring heights in preference. The low land rarely escapes entirely, but is less affected as a general rule than the overlooking hill.

Leaving the plain, Dr. Williams next seeks further illustration of his position on the high lands. " The different force" (he says) " by which the paludal poison is attracted by different surfaces, has been often observed in the West Indies. Fort Hildane, at Porto Maria, (Jamaica), occupies the extreme point of a promontory, which projects considerably from the main-land and divides the bay into two basin-like recesses. This promontory, which is one hundred and fifty feet above the level of the sea, and two hundred feet across, is so nearly *perpendicular* and so nearly alike in all its faces, that it has the appearance of an artificial structure, raised for the defence of the harbor. It is formed of pure carbonate of lime, and on looking at it merely as a dry mass of chalk, washed on three sides by the sea, we should imagine it to be one of the healthiest situations in the West Indies. Two streams, however, fall into the bay, one on each side of this headland at about a quarter of a mile distant. They move slowly, and their banks are covered with Mangrove, which it is presumed furnishes the more palpable cause of fever. But it is remarkable that the inhabitants of Porto Maria, which is situated on either side of one of these streams, do not appear to suffer from their position, while at Fort Hildane, the returns of the sick have shown it to be productive of a fever so deadly, that for some years past the Fort has not been garrisoned."

He relates another parallel instance, viz: at Port Spain, the Capital of Trinidad, where the town, on the marshy lowlands, is infinitely more healthy than " the covering heights, which rise out of one extremity of the marsh, and which are composed of the dryest and most healthy materials, or pure lime stone." * * * " No portion of their diversified surface, however elevated, sunken, or walled round, has been a security from the exhalations below."

Dr. Fergusson, in his oft quoted paper on Malaria, in vol. 9 of the "Transactions of the Royal Society of Edinburgh," adds his high authority to the support of these opinions. He says—" Another proof that from the attraction above mentioned, it (Malaria) *creeps along the ground,* so as to concentrate and collect on the sides of the adjacent hills, instead of floating directly upwards in the atmosphere, is the *remarkable fact that it is certainly absorbed by passing over a small surface of water.*"

Fergusson testifies also, as do writers on diseases of hot climates generally, to the fact that Malaria is more concentrated near the ground, and consequently a much larger proportion of persons are attacked in a first than a second, and in a second than a third story; thus proving that Malaria, in *some* of its forms at least, keeps itself *near the ground.*

The " *altitudinal range*" of Malaria is a point of endless confusion; facts the most contradictory are presented to us in profusion by our highest authorities. All fevers, however different their habitudes and habitats, are thrown together, pell mell, and set down to one common morbific cause.

How are these contradictions to be reconciled? From the facts given, and many others which are easily produced, it would seem that Yellow Fever and Intermittent fevers are governed by very different laws in this respect. It must be admitted, for example, that if the *materies morbi* of Yellow Fever does not (as Fergusson says) " *creep along the ground*" like a worm, we have evidence of its existence only very *near the ground.* We have numerous examples in the West Indies, of its attacking ground floors of barracks, while the third story was almost exempt, and the truth of the fact is familiar to the profession in our Southern towns. But can the same admission be made for Intermittent Fever? There can be no doubt that ground floors, from their dampness, from various impure vapors and gases arising from the earth's surface, as also from imperfect ventilation, are unwholesome; but I am by no means satisfied that the specific poison which produces Intermittent, exists in greater force near the surface of the earth than higher up. A patient, debilitated and disordered by the causes just enumerated, might become more susceptible to the impression of this, as to other morbid poisons, and thus give support to the idea that the poison really exists here in greater force. But there is another explanation for the fact which is more satisfactory, viz: Intermittent is a disease of the country and not of the towns, and the houses out of town are almost always surrounded by trees which we are told obstruct the progress of Malaria. They are usually of a height to protect upper stories, while the winds blow without obstruction under the foliage, and may thus conduct Malaria to the lower floors. My own observation, in South Carolina and Alabama, which is by no means limited, satisfies me that lower stories have little advantage as regards *Intermittents,* though when *very near* the ground are insalubrious *in* and *out* of the region of periodic fevers. Macculloch and the other authors give us numerous instances, where Intermittents have selected *in preference upper stories,* while the *lower ones were left exempt.* The fact, too, is notorious that the summit of a hill, however precipitous, may be its sides, even a lime rock 150 or 200 feet high, as at Fort Hildane and Porto Maria, is more liable to Intermittents than the low land and marshes, which it overlooks. By what unknown power can a rock thus draw up this Malaria from a depth of 200 feet? The simple affinity of lime for moisture is inadequate to this effect, and still less when we come to elevations of 1000 or more feet.

Fergusson furnishes us with the following curious and instructive statement :

"In the Island of Antigua, the same results were confirmed in a striking manner. The autumn of 1816 became very sickly, and Yellow Fever broke out in all its low marshy quarters, while the milder *Remittent pervaded the island generally.* The British garrison of English Harbor soon felt the influence of that unwholesome place. They were distributed on a range of fortified hills that surround the dock-yard. The principal of these, Monk's Hill, at the bottom of the bay, rises perpendicular above the marshes to the height of 600 feet. The other garrisoned hill, which goes by the name of the Ridge, is about 100 feet lower, but instead of rising perpendicularly, it slopes backwards from the swamps of English Harbor. It was the duty of the white troops, in both these forts, to take the guards and duties of the dockyards amongst the marshes below, and so pestiferous was their atmosphere, that it often occurred to a well seasoned soldier, mounting the night guard in perfect health, to be seized with furious delirium while standing sentry, and when carried back to the barracks, on Monk's Hill, to expire in all the horrors of Black Vomit within less than thirty hours from the first attack ; but during all this, not a single case of Yellow Fever, nor fever of any kind, occurred to the inhabitants of Monk's Hill; that is to say, the garrison staff, the superior officers, the women, the drummers, &c., all in fact that were not obliged to *sleep* out of the garrison, or take the duties below, remained in perfect health. The result on the Ridge was not quite the same, but it was equally curious and instructive. The artillery soldiers (17 in number) never took any of the night guards, but they occupied a barrack about 300 feet above the marshes, not perpendicular above them, like Monk's Hill, but a little retired. Not a case of Yellow Fever or Black Vomit occurred amongst them, but every man, without a single exception, suffered an attack of the ordinary Remittent, of which one of them died ; and at the barrack on the top of the Ridge, at the height of 500 feet, and still farther retired from the marshes, there scarcely occurred any fever worthy of notice."

These and similar facts are brought forward by Fergusson and others to prove the identity of these different types of Fever—they say that the concentrated poison which produces Yellow fever below, in rising to the hill, becomes so diluted as to produce only the milder forms of paludal fever. This explanation is untenable, because it is a general law of intermittent and remittent fevers that they every where affect, more the hills than the lowland from which they emanate, not only in Yellow fever localities, but in those regions *where Yellow fever is unknown.* I have shown elsewhere that yellow fever is a disease of towns, and intermittents of the country, and that yellow fever occurs, (as at Barbadoes) where intermittents do not : and that if *dilution* of the poison had anything to do with the matter, the winds blowing over points infected with yellow fever should strew intermittents before them.

Even Fergusson with all his talent, learning and industry, by taking a false position, has involved himself in the same inconsistencies as other writers on Malaria. In the very article I have been quoting from, he says: "In selecting situations for ports and barracks, it had been observed with surprise, that the border and even the centre of the marsh, proved a less dangerous quarter than the *neighboring heights* of the purest soil and healthiest temperature; and this has never been more strongly exemplified than in the instances I am going to relate." He then goes on to relate the instance already alluded to of Port Spain, Trinidad—where the heights overlook the town. He says—" no place however elevated, or sunk, or sheltered, or walled in, gives security against the exhalations from below, only it *has been distinctly ascertained, that these prevail with more or less malignity, exactly in proportion to the elevation of the dwelling.* The lower, consequently the *nearer. the marsh,* the better. The tops of the ridges are uninhabitable—on the highest point, at an elevation of 400 feet, and farther removed from the marsh than the town itself, a large martello tower was built to defend the place. It possessed a fine temperature, but proved so dangerous that it was obliged to be abandoned; not even a creole mulatto Spaniard could sleep in it with impunity for a single night, after a course of dry weather."

In what an awful fog do these statements leave us! At one moment the poison gets *weaker* as it *goes* up; and the next, it becomes *concentrated* in the same ratio as you come down!

These strange and apparently whimsical habits of the morbific cause of Paludal Fevers would seem to corroborate the opinion that it is not governed by the motions of the atmosphere, and that it is more under the control of some *mysterious instinct.* In 1842 and '43, when yellow fever was progressing literally at a snail's pace, through the town which was constantly swept by the sea or land breezes, I confidently advised persons *out of the infected district,* to leave town, before the disease reached them, and seek safety in the country. Those who took the advice escaped, while those in their vicinity who remained, were reached and many attacked by the yellow fever.

Dr. Williams, in his chapter on "the Paludal Poison," after detailing a number of curious facts illustrative of the *Altitudinal* and *Horizontal range* of Malaria, says:—"The preceding facts are sufficient to show, if the altitude to which the paludal poison ascends, greatly varies in different places, its horizontal spread also varies according to the surface over which it passes, being strongly attracted by some bodies and altogether without affinity for others. In attempting to assign the law which may explain these varying, and often apparently opposite phenomena, there is no hypothesis so satisfactory as that which supposes the paludal poison to follow the same laws as those which govern the vapor or dew, by which it is held either in a state of solution or suspension, and which may be generalized as follows, &c."

He then branches off on the theory of dews—tells us of the radiating, reflecting, attracting and absorbing properties of different plants, soils, rocks, &c., accounts for the fevers on the hills at Porto Maria and Port Spain by the affinity of the *lime* rocks for moisture—explains the influence of water over malaria by its power of condensing the dews when it is colder than the air, and by its repelling the dews under the opposite circumstances by throwing off vapor from its surface. In short, Dr.

Williams and others have not only exhausted all the known laws of dews in sustaining their hypothesis, but have resorted to many forced constructions, and yet all falls far short of being satisfactory.

His recapitulation of the theory of dews is by no means well done, and I therefore prefer giving the established facts in my own way. The instructive little work of Griffiths on the " Chemistry of the four Seasons" presents us with some very clear illustrations of several of the points, which may be quoted with advantage. " It is an old saying that the *hills draw the wet,* or " *hills draw the clouds,*" but they have no inherent or particular attraction in this respect ; they *are only surfaces of the earth projecting above its common level.*" In this he is unquestionably correct,—there can be no " inherent or particular attraction" in a part of the same soil merely because it has been thrown up 50 or 500 feet above another portion—the difference of height is often too trivial for any appreciable Barometrical change which could influence the *elevation of vapors ;* and the appearance of marsh fevers on elevations cannot be accounted for on the supposition of attraction of soils in moisture (as the lime hills spoken of), because it is notorious in our Southern States that the composition of the hill is immaterial ;—wherever the morbific cause of intermittents is generated in the valley, the exposed hill which overlooks it, is attacked whether it be sand, clay, lime, rich dark vegetable mould, &c. ; the color too, as white, black, red, gray, &c., makes little if any difference.

Lime certainly has a greater affinity for moisture than clay or sand ; and yet so far from its being true that hills of this composition precipitate more moisture than the valley, the reverse will usually be found true. It is well known that plants, as grass, grains, cotton, trees, &c., and the rich *black* soils of the swamps are the best radiators of heat and consequently the best condensors of moisture. It is therefore in the luxuriant valleys, and not on the light colored hill, that we should expect, and really do find, the heavy dews.

" If, " says Mr. Griffith," the thermometer be placed on a grass-plat, it will very frequently indicate a temperature of 15 or 20 degrees colder, than one suspended over the grass at the height of 3 or 4 feet—thus proving that radiation is proceeding with extreme rapidity in the one case from the comparatively solid vegetable and soil, but not from the ambient air." Accordingly, the portions of air in immediate contact with the grass, become much colder than those far above, and are compelled to deposit dew ; and if the air over a green locality remain tranquil for some hours, this phenomenon will solely ensue from the lower and colder portions."

" Small valleys and hollow ways, permit the air to remain undisturbed ; and although they are apparently situations sheltered from cold, yet they are frequently more subject to reduction of temperature than higher situations, and accordingly, much to our surprise, we find delicate plants chilled or even frost bitten in hollows, whilst others suffer no injury upon the adjacent slopes."

How common is it in autumn when we look out upon a meadow or corn field, to see a dense white mist only a few feet in height directly incumbent on the surface, whilst the air is clear and bright above with the rays of the sun. Or we may even walk through the field with the lower part of the body enveloped in the mist, whilst the upper is free from its humidity.

There would then seem to be no known law of *dews*, or any other by which malaria can be transferred in a more concentrated form from the valley to a great elevation. It is evident from the facts given that if the poison be entangled with vapor, it should be most concentrated where the dews are heaviest, viz : on the dark, rich soil of the valley, covered with vegetation and not on the barren hill top. If, too, it be true that the malaria is entangled with dew, it is difficult to imagine how it should be so much more active at night—how does it rise up from the valley and ascend to the mountain summit 1000 or more feet (of which we have examples) at a time when the vapors not only cease to rise from the earth, but are rapidly *depositing* on the cold surface of the lowland ?

It has been said that the malaria is active only at night-fall when the dews first descend and in the morning when they again are called up by the sun. But this is not true for several good reasons—1st. Malaria is often generated on a very small spot of ground, and the emanations which arise from this like the smoke from the chimneys must necessarily be borne off to the distance of several miles, and would not descend upon the overhanging hill as at Port Spain, or Porto Maria—2nd. Instances are common where persons have contracted fevers by going during the night to the infected district—as in the cases mentioned of the sentries at English Harbor—those travelling through the Pontrine marshes at night, &c. It is a familiar fact in Charleston, South Carolina, that it is hazardous for persons to leave the city and go into the neighboring marsh lands at night; and the danger is greatly increased if they allow themselves to fall asleep—instances might easily be multiplied. It is worthy of remark, too, that when the cool nights of autumn arrive, the morbific cause seems to attain its greatest virulence, though the valley from the increasing coldness of its surface, greatly increases in its power of condensing moisture, and it need hardly be said that a surface cannot condense and throw off aqueous vapor at the same time. So marked is this phenomenon, that we often see repeated light frosts in the valley and even thin sheets of ice on the ground, while the thermometer a few feet above in the air does not fall below 40 degrees of Fahrenheit—at the same time the hills are entirely exempt from the frosts and their vegetation remains untouched.

As far as we have any means of judging, all emanations are more concentrated as we approach the focus whence they originate, and if there is any analogy between these and Malaria, its greatest concentration should be in the valley. It is not on the hill, but in the marsh that our olfactories are offended by its putrid odors; so is it with putrid animal matter, and odors of every description. In the interior of South Carolina, away from the influence of the sea breeze, the nights are usually very calm and sultry—far more so than in the prairies of the West; and we should here expect (according to the theory we are combatting), that near the rivers and in small valleys where the fogs lie near and on the surface undisturbed during the autumn, the poison should produce its deadliest effects; but the hill here too suffers more than the valley. The idea that the hill suffers most, because the currents of air cause the fogs to *infringe on the hills* is alike untenable ;

a wind rolling along this heavy mass of fog over a wide plain, and bearing it up to the top of a hill, could not certainly render it more concentrated.

It would certainly be quite as philosophical (as the Malarial theory) to suppose that some insect or animalcule, hatched in the lowlands, like the musquito, after passing through its metamorphoses, takes flight, and either from preference for a different atmosphere, or impelled by one of those extraordinary instincts which many are known to possess, wings its way to the hill top to fulfil its appointed destiny.

6th. "Experience has proved, that in cities where Yellow Fever prevails, the places which are low, pent up, and badly ventilated, such as narrow streets, alleys, cul de sacs, first and second stories, &c., are the places most dangerous to inhabit—observation has shown that it is the same with intermittent fevers."

I must here join issue again with M. Chervin, and feel confident that every physician of observation in these diseases, from Boston to New Orleans, will sustain me in a denial of this conclusion. All observation and all facts contradict it. Yellow Fever is a disease of the towns and Intermittents of the country. The City of Charleston stands in the midst of a very pestiferous region, where all the grades of periodic fevers prevail, but no Yellow Fever. Since the town was built a new local atmosphere has been engendered which has expelled the periodic fevers, and introduced the *new disease, Yellow Fever.* The experience of the whole world proves that whenever a large town is built Intermittent is expelled from the soil, though it may still hang about the outskirts. Even in Rome, which is surrounded by one of the most poisonous miasmatic regions in Europe, Sir James Johnson, in his "*Change of Air*," tells us, "The low, crowded, and abominably filthy quarter of the Jews, on the banks of the Tiber, near the foot of the Capitol, may probably owe its acknowledged freedom from the fatal Malaria, to its sheltered site and inconceivably dense population."

An *Epidemic* of periodic fevers, in a large town, is a thing unheard of. The bills of mortality of Charleston, Mobile, and New Orleans will show that when these cities escape Yellow Fever, they never have Epidemics of other fevers.

7th. "It is a well known fact that the miasms which produce periodic fevers, are infinitely more active in the night than the day. Those which give birth to Yellow Fever possess likewise extraordinary power of action when the sun is below the horizon."

The concession, were we to yield this point, would be unimportant in establishing the identity of these diseases. At all events, much that we have already said so far disproves the position as to make but a few more words necessary, in reference to it. Though fully aware of the opinions generally expressed to the contrary by writers, I am by no means sure that a difference does not here exist between the two diseases. The Campagna, the Maremma and the Pontines we are told may be traversed with impunity during the day, and many facts are given of the same nature in relation to Yellow Fever; but I am satisfied that persons often take Yellow Fever by coming into Mobile during the day for an hour or two, though the risk is certainly much greater at night.

A strangely absurd reason is frequently assigned for the increased activity of the morbific cause of Yellow Fever at night. It is said that the poison is volatilized by the heat of the sun during the day, and being entangled with aqueous vapor, is precipitated with the dews of evening in a condensed form. Not a particle of proof is given to sustain this assumption, which is contradicted by well known facts. In Charleston, for example, where Yellow Fever occurs, while periodic fevers prevail for many miles around, the facts would be reversed. The town and country are almost incessantly swept by the land and sea breezes, and at night the vapor from the marshes of the country should fall on the town, and produce " country fevers," while the Yellow Fever emanations would fall at some distant point in the country. The Yellow Fever sometimes is so circumscribed as to be confined to a single alley or very small portion of the city.

All the attempts heretofore made to account for the greater activity of the morbific cause of Yellow Fever at night have failed, and in my humble opinion the fact may be much better explained by a reference to habits of Insect Life. Many of the Infusoria, as well as insects proper, are rendered inactive by too much light, heat, or dryness. They remain quiet through the day, and do their work at night. This fact is too familiar to require illustration. The moth tribe, the night musquitoes, many of the Aphides, &c., are familiar examples.

8th. " In the Equinoxial regions, Yellow Fever attacks in general, almost exclusively, unacclimated persons; intermittent and remittent fevers attack also in preference (though M. Gerardin has advanced the contrary opinion in this assembly) those subjects who come from a healthy into marshy countries."*

9th. " Yellow Fever attacks particularly strong and vigorous men, who pass from northern to southern climates ; it is the same with intermittents and remittents, as is abundantly proved by the successive occupations of Italy, Spain, the Ionian Isles, Morea, and Algiers, by our troops."

It is true that Yellow Fever attacks almost exclusively the unacclimated, and selects in preference the robust natives of cold regions, but I have strong reasons for believing that M. Gerardin is correct in denying the applicability of this rule to periodic fevers. Such persons, in consequence of their sanguineous temperaments, are more apt when attacked, to suffer severely than the natives of hot climates ; but they are not more liable, if so much, as the latter to take these diseases. No population can ever be acclimated against periodic fevers, and the fact is equally certain that every attack of Intermittent increases the susceptibility to others. There is no place in the United States where the population can become acclimated against " marsh fevers." While the acclimated population of Charleston are living (as I have shown by the bills of mortality) in greater health than that of any large town in this country, the inhabitants of the surrounding country suffer from all the horrors of miasmatic fevers, and present all the physical signs of an enfeebled, degenerate race. Go to the Campagna, the Maremma, the Pontines—even to the " Eternal City itself—and ask for the de-

---

* The pamphlet from which I quote is a report of M. Chervin, read before the Acadamic Royale de medicine in 1842—page 120.

scendants of the proud Romans, who, two thousand years ago, held the world in bondage ! The ghastly picture of the population drawn then by Cicero and Horace, has only become more hideous with time. The miserable inhabitants are now, even more than then, skulking from the fatal Malaria, and hiding themselves on the mountain tops and in the crevices of the rocks ; and the jaundiced skin, the bloated abdomen and withered limbs point to the physical degeneracy of the race.

If there are apparent exceptions, in some parts of the world, to the above facts, it is probably only because different forms of fever have been unproperly attributed to one cause ; but the face of the globe cannot show an exception, where genuine Intermittent fever prevails.

We may refer in illustration of this point to Fergusson and the other army and navy surgeons who have written on the diseases of the Peninsular War, and whose statements, in some particulars, seem to conflict with opinions advanced by me. They mention instances where the troops suffered much more than the natives, a result reasonably to have been expected, even if their susceptibilities were equal, when we take into consideration the exposure—sleeping on the ground, and various hardships which they endured. The facts given below are sufficient to excite strong doubts as to the *identity* of the diseases with which the troops and natives suffered. All the descriptions of those fevers I have seen are incomplete and unsatisfactory.

Mr. Fergusson, in his admirable paper on *Marsh Poison*, before alluded to, amongst other interesting particulars, give the following : The English troops, after the battle of Talevera, retreated into the " dry, sandy, rocky plains" of Estramadura, " at a time when the country was so dry and arid for want of rain that the Guadiana River itself and all the smaller streams had in fact *ceased to be streams*, and were no more than lines of detached pools in the courses that had formerly been rivers ; and there they suffered from Remittent fevers of such destructive malignity, that the enemy and all Europe believed that the English host was extirpated ; and the superstitious natives, *though sickly themselves*, unable to account for disease of such *uncommon type amongst the strangers*, declared they had all been poisoned by eating the mushrooms which spring up after the autumnal rains, about the time the Epidemic had attained its height. The aggravated cases of the disease differed little or nothing from the *worst Yellow Fever of the West Indies.*"

The English army surgeons present us many other facts of similar import, and the well known habits of the fevers of our Southern States would lead to the conclusion that Fergusson, as in the Case of Antigua before spoken of, confounds distinct diseases. A camp disease of obscure origin was probably generated, different from the paludal fever of the natives, who were from long residence in the climate proof against this malady which " differed little or nothing from the worst *Yellow Fever* of the West Indies." The same astonishment was probably expressed by the Aborigines of the West Indies when the foreigners were first swept off before their eyes with Yellow Fever—a disease to them of " uncommon type."

Fergusson tells us, too, that the Estramadura fevers occurred in a season and locality, where the extreme dryness of the sandy soil and the paucity of vegetable matter precluded all idea of vegetable matter being a cause. Vegetable matter is *certainly* not a cause of Yellow Fever ; and I do not see how any one who would travel through the alluvial country of Louisiana, where all the causes of Intermittents exist in the highest possible degree *without these diseases*, and then follow through the chain of facts in this paper, can have any *settled belief* in vegetable decomposition as a cause of Periodic Fevers. When I speak of "all the causes of Intermittents" I mean those usually assigned as rich soil, vegetable matter, stagnant matter, both wild and cultivated lands, hot climate &c. ; all that the malarial "hypothesis" could possibly ask, is here in profusion, but *no fever;* while the "dry, rocky, sandy" desert of Estramadura is uninhabitable, at least to foreigners, and the natives are also sickly.

10th. " The individual who has contracted an Intermittent Fever in a marshy place, attenuates the effect of the poison and hastens his recovery by going to reside in a healthy locality; the same thing happens with the Yellow Fever, but in a less marked manner, because in this case the paludal ." *intoxication*" is more rapid and is carried to a higher degree."

There is certainly no parallelism between the cases here ; but on the contrary the most marked contrast. The poison of Intermittent Fever is so *adhesive* that the London writers tell us, that persons returning to that city (where Intermittent is *unknown*) with seeds of the disease contracted in the West Indies, will continue to *relapse for twenty years.* In spite, too, of travel, mineral waters and all other remedies, Periodic Fevers will often leave enlargement of the spleen, disorders of the liver, dyspepsia and other chronic affections to haunt the victim for life. How different is it with Yellow Fever? Like Roderick Dhu, it scorns all unfair advantage and nobly "tries the quarrel hilt to hilt," and when the "dubious strife" is over, if his antagonist has proved the victor, he may "falter thanks to heaven for life redeemed, and rise unmolested by the "*foeman's Clan.*"

There are rarely sequelæ to Yellow Fever, and strange as the assertion may seem to those unacquainted with this disease, I have seen more cases of dyspepsia cured by attacks of it than by all the doctors of my acquaintance.

The last part of the above quotation is equally erroneous ;—there is no evidence that the poisoning in Yellow Fever "is more rapid and carried to a higher degree" than in other forms of what are termed "paludal fevers." The high grades of bilious and congestive fevers are quite as rapid—as unmanageable and fatal as the most malignant forms of Yellow Fever. In the interior of our South Western States, where Yellow Fever is unknown, these fatal forms abound—often causing death in a few hours.

11th. " Finally all the differential signs which are said to exist between Yellow and Remittent Bilious Fevers of hot climates are absolutely without foundation, such as the appearance of the eyes, nature and seat of the pain in the head, absence of remission, color of the skin, duration of the disease, morbid state of the stomach—nature of the matters vomited, immunity produced by a first attack, mode of treatment &c.

If a light remittent fever be compared with a very intense Yellow Fever, we shall without doubt see very marked differences in the symptoms of the two affections ; but if we put beside a severe remittent a mild case of Yellow Fever, we shall see none ; for as remarks Doctor Repey : " There is a point where these fevers are so confounded, that they really become one and the same disease," the same affection under different forms and various degrees."

When a writer starts in a wrong direction, the farther he goes, the farther does he wander from the path of truth. Such I fear has been the case with our " estimable ami " Monsieur Chervin (with whom, by the by, we had the pleasure of a personal acquaintance) and we must say of him as he said of Rochoux : " il a observé la fièvre jaune assez long temps pour la bien connoître, mais malheureusement il l'a vue avec une opinion préconçue"—and I cannot help thinking he would have come to very different conclusions had he, as I have done, sat down quietly in one place and studied Yellow Fever through all its grades and changes, instead of running incessantly from place to place for eight years in search of facts. It would at first glance seem a matter of surprise that one who has sacrificed so much time in the cause, and who has written so well on the point of Contagion, should have so erred on other points ; but a moment's reflection should satisfy us that by the course he adopted he necessarily had to take the testimony of others (most of whom were *not observers*) instead of observing for himself.

We have no space here to follow out the line of demarcation between the two diseases by comparing their Pathology and Symptomatology, and must rely principally on the difference of habits &c. already treated of. Diagnosis, between two diseases, even the most opposite in their causes and nature, is often embarrassing ; but how much more difficult is it to lay down conclusive diagnostic signs between diseases of the same genus, though different species. If a physician were called in the forming stage of a number of cases of Plague, Small Pox, Yellow Fever, some forms of Typhus, and other diseases arising from Morbid Poisons, as well as certain vegetable poisons, he would be much at a loss how to distinguish them for two or three days ; and in some of those in which the characteristic signs are never developed (as Small Pox without eruption &c.), a diagnosis never could be made. It should not be wondered at then, that difficulty of diagnosis should sometimes occur between Bilious and Yellow Fevers, which belong to the same family, the same season and same locality.

Another strong reason for this difficulty of diagnosis is found in the fact that no two Epidemic or atmospheric diseases can possibly prevail together without becoming blended. When Yellow Fever prevails, as I have seen it, in a milder form than what we term Epidemic, it is invariably seen more or less blended with the Intermittents and Remittents of the environs—they are mingled in every possible grade. Andral, in speaking of the influence of Epidemics over other diseases, makes the following pertinent remarks.

" But on all these diseases, differing in their seat, it impresses a uniform modification ; it brings them to an *identity* of nature, and consequently an identity of treatment. It is therefore much less important in therapeutics to know the seat even of a disease than the " *Epidemic Constitution*," under which it has taken birth ; for it is on this constitution that the treatment should be based." He goes on to illustrate, by giving instances of the "Inflammatory Constitution," the Bilious Constitution, the Mucous or Catarrhal Constitution, the Putrid &c., during which a Pneumonia or other inflammatory disease would require "the most *opposite treatment.*"

I, on a former occasion, explained more fully the nature of those cases which are termed Intermittent and Remittent Yellow Fever. In 1844 many of these cases occurred in Mobile—in this year there were only 40 deaths from Yellow Fever and no *Epidemic Constitution* of the atmosphere was established—the two diseases struggling for mastery, with nearly equal force, were blended in every conceivable degree in different subjects—sometimes the Periodic and at others the true Yellow Fever type predominating—the periodic type preponderating particularly in the suburbs, near the marshes. The cases were sprinkled over the whole town without being confined to any particular focus.

No one at all familiar with the history of Epidemics could doubt this tendency of diseases to amalgamation; if there should perchance be a Sceptic, let him wade through the four volumes of Ozanam "des maladies Epidemiques," and the facts will bring him to the conclusion which reason points to.

Suppose a Rattlesnake or a Tarantula were to bite a patient laboring under Intermittent Fever, or he should swallow a large dose of vegetable poison—what would probably follow? The effects of the two poisons would be blended, and the stronger would predominate over the weaker—after the subsidence of the effect of the newly applied poison, if the patient survive, should we be surprised to see the Intermittent recur and resume its regular course? Ozanam tells us that when Small Pox is prevailing in the East, the plague will sometimes come and drive it from the field. After a certain time a few scattering cases of the dormant Small Pox reappear, and this is looked upon as a sure sign of disappearance of the Plague, and the Small Pox about to resume its course. Williams in his "*Morbid Poisons*" says—"The variolous poison is capable of coexisting with many other poisons; also of influencing their actions and being reciprocally influenced by them.— Dessessarz has seen Variolæ coexist with Scarlatina and with hooping cough; Cruikshanks, with Measles; Frank, with Psora; Dimsdale, with Syphilis; and Heberden, with Intermittent Fever, who adds in his commentaries a case of this latter complication lately occurred in St. Thomas's Hospital. A patient was admitted laboring under tertian fever, which was unusually intractable and resisted quinine. At length, however, the variolæ appeared and the fever subsided; but no sooner had the eruption run its course, than the intermittent again appeared and was now readily cured by the usual means. Ring even mentions a case of triple disease coexisting, or of the Small Pox, the Measles and the hooping cough, all of which ran their course together."—It is needless to multiply facts on this point as they may be found in the works of Williams, Ozanam and other writers on Epidemic diseases.

In short, what is our whole system of Therapeutics based on, but the modifying influence which one impression on the system exerts over another. Why do we give mercury to cure Syphilis—quinine to cure Intermittent, &c., unless to counteract the action of one poison by that of another impression. Why are we so cautious in selecting a proper time for administering opium and other drugs. In a word, it is evident that the skill of the physician depends entirely upon a proper selection of modifying agents and time for their administration.

The subject of *Morbid Poisons* is one of incomprehensible difficulties. Epidemic diseases, as Influenza, Measles, Scarlet Fever, Small-Pox, Hooping-cough, &c., often prevail so together, or follow each other in such a mysterious manner, that some writers, as Holland and others, have suggested a common morbific cause, variously modified by season, climate, meteorological changes, temperaments, &c. &c. This opinion has not gained much favor with the profession ; but the *fact* stands, that diseases which are regarded as the most opposite in their causes, symptoms, pathology and duration, are sometimes strangely allied.

A singular instance has twice occurred in Mobile during the last few years—viz: an amalgamation of Measles and Scarlet Fever—I have seen in the same house (as have other physicians) a case of pure measles, another of pure Scarlet fever, and a third in which the symptoms of the two were so commingled as to render it impossible to say which predominated—these mixed cases commenced with all the symptoms of measles, as inflammation of the eyes, catarrhal symptoms, sneezing, distinct measly rash, &c.; and in a few days a putrid sore throat, and scarlet fever tongue would appear, and if the patient survived, all the sequelæ of Scarlet fever, as affections of the ears, extensive desquamation, dropsical effusions, &c. It is very remarkable that some of these cases were still farther complicated by distinct chicken pox, thus showing a co-existence of three diseases generally regarded as distinct.

When Yellow Fever shakes off its mild endemic form and assumes that of a great *Epidemic,* as it did here in 1839, it comes robed in majesty and power—all febrile diseases disappear before it, or are compelled to wear its livery—the peculiar characteristics of the disease stand out boldly, and with few exceptions, all difficulty of diagnosis vanishes—patients are stricken down by hundreds with attacks varying from the mildest to the most malignant and yet all wholly unlike periodic fevers—in the same family and house, one will be so lightly attacked as scarcely to lie down, while another is dying with all the horrors of black-vomit; and what is particularly worthy of note, the light cases pass off spontaneously in two or three days *without a dose of quinine,* and afford *protection against the disease in after years.*

We are led to conclude from the mass of evidence on this point, that yellow fever varies much as to type in different localities—in extremely hot climates for example, as in Asia and Africa, the excitement is more intense, and the brain is more uniformly and violently affected. It is well known that every morbid poison influences different individuals in very different degrees—a familiar illustration may be seen in the degrees of violence presented by Scarlet Fever, Small-pox, Typhus, &c., where persons have been equally exposed to the morbific causes. The same variety is seen amongst the cases of yellow fever. One will, as we have already said, have it very mildly, while another will be struck down speechless, as by appoplexy, and die in a few hours. Yet there is quite as much uniformity in the symptoms of yellow fever as in other diseases arising from morbid poisons. Leaving however what may be called anomalous cases, the disease is every where in its pure form, characterized as a *fever of one paroxysm.* The following is the ordinary type of the disease in Mobile. The subject while in perfect health is seized with a slight chilly sensation which occurs either during the day in the midst of his avocations, or he is awakened by it at night during a profound natural sleep—acceleration⸴ of pulse to 100, to 110 or 115 beats in a minute soon follows, accompanied by *moderate thirst,* and most excruciating pains in the head, back, and limbs—the acceleration of pulse and thirst are not at all in proportion to the violence of the pains and general anxiety—often the pulse during the fever does not exceed 90 and the skin is of natural temperature and perspiring all the while.— After about 40 hours the fever subsides and the patient is left in a state of calm, called by some a *remission,* during which there is frequently such a complete absence of all external signs of disease, that a physician unaccustomed to yellow fever, would not hesitate to pronounce the patient out of danger and convalescent. This calm lasts another 40 hours, and is followed by the stage of collapse in which there seems to be a sudden and almost complete exhaustion of the vital powers—during this last stage the patient usually requires stimulants, such as brandy, porter, &c., and if he does not sink with or without black-vomit, the disease *runs its course,* and by the 6th or 7th day, he enters fairly into convalescence. There is no fever after the first paroxysm, unless the lesion of some organ again calls the heart into action—a second fever is not a *necessary part of the disease.* Another striking peculiarity of yellow fever, too, is the entire absence of bilious vomiting after the paroxysm of fever has passed—if perchance you see a blue, green, or yellow tinge in the clear fluid vomited, you may hail it as the harbinger of safety—the prognosis is almost certain. Contrast these symptoms with those of bilious fever,—each in its distinct uncomplicated form, and where I would ask is the *identity* of which M. Chervin speaks?

In 1839 Yellow Fever in Mobile assumed its highest *Epidemic* form —it not only overwhelmed the town, but, gathering extraordinary strength (like the Cholera) it burst over its accustomed bounds and ravaged the habitations around for several miles. There was something, I presume, peculiarly favorable to the generation of its morbific cause this season, for it occurred in violent form in nearly all the towns on the Gulf of Mexico.

Admitting, as has been argued, that genuine Yellow Fever does occasionally present the Intermittent type, with a succession of paroxysms, the fact would deserve little weight in settling the question of identity. *Intermittence* is an unexplained pathological fact when connected with any disease. Many diseases, in opposition to their ordinary phenomena, may assume the intermittent type—as Neuralgia, Opthalmia, Paralysis, etc. Even Pleurisies, Pneumonias and other inflammatory disorders, in our latitude, frequently assume the bilious remitting form. What are termed Bilious Pneumonia and Bilious Pleurisy, are Phlegmasiæ proper, modified by the morbific cause (Malaria) of Periodic fever.

It was not my plan to argue the Insect origin of Periodic fevers in this paper, but the morbific causes of Fevers have been so long and so inseparably united in the minds of the profession that it is almost impossible to tear them asunder now.

All writers are agreed on the fact that a very imperfect barrier will obstruct the progress of *marsh miasmata*—a row of houses or of trees, etc., will often effectally protect dwellings from the access of this fatal poison. It is moreover asserted that these miasms are not only impeded, but *attracted* by trees, and this would seem to be the case from the well known fact that the danger is greater from sleeping in a cluster of trees, than in an open space.

I have been able, in my researches, to discover no facts of this kind in connection with Yellow Fever, and my personal observation repudiates them *in toto*. We never find Yellow fever as the Sportsman say "up a tree," but on the contrary, the *materies morbi*, whatever it be, creeps along the ground, regardless of winds, passing under and through houses, trees, etc., and knowing no impediment but a sheet of water.*

The Insect theory is perhaps as applicable to Periodic as Yellow Fever. We can well understand how Insects wafted by the winds (as happens with musquitoes, flying ants, many of the Aphides, etc.,) should haul up on the first tree, house or other object in their course, offering a resting place ; but no one can imagine how a gas or emanation, entangled or not with aqueous vapor, while sweeping along on the wings of the wind, could be caught in this way ; and we, on the contrary, often see fogs and clouds swept by winds *through the forest.* Another insuperable difficulty, too, is found in the fact that the dews are deposited as heavily on the one side as on the other of the protecting woods. I have very strongly impressed on my memory an instance of this kind : at my father's summer residence in South Carolina, our house stood upon a hill which gradually declined for half a mile till it terminated in the lowlands of the plantation ; a row of trees, which were so scattered as but imperfectly to obstruct the view of the fields below, stood about midway between the latter and the residence ; though the fact was inexplicable, this imperfect barrier *did* protect us, and our family lived there for fourteen summers, with uninterrupted health. The trees presented scarcely any impediment to the force of the winds, and *I never saw heavier dews than those on the rich grass plat around the house.* After my father's death, the old residence fell into the hands of my brother-in law, and the protecting row of trees having been cut down, it has become so subject to marsh fevers, that he has been compelled to abandon it.

If these emanations are *attracted* by and attached to trees, how do they get loose again and come down to attack persons in *lower stories?*

They should remain on the trees until again evaporated by the morning's sun—these miasms must have some power *per se* of migrating, and clustering in trees, else these facts could not exist. It should be borne in mind, too, that the very writers who thus run their Malaria up trees, are those who tell us that its specific gravity is so great that it lies on the ground ! !

---

* It is a curious fact that from 1829 to 1837 there was no Epidemic of Yellow Fever in Mobile. and during this time the streets were beautifully shelled ; since '37 we have had it five times, and the shelling was not continued. If the Insect theory be correct, could the lime be an impediment to their progress across streets ?

CONTAGION.

If by this term we understand that a morbid poison generated in one living body may by contact, either mediate or immediate, reproduce an identical disease in another, then are we justified in denying that Yellow Fever is a contagious disease. But while without hesitation I take this position, I am equally strong in the conviction that there exists no conclusive evidence, that the germ or *materies morbi* may not be transported from one locality to another. There are many curious facts connected with this question which require a passing notice.

The Insect theory here again comes to our aid, and may explain difficulties which have much perplexed writers on contagion. The early history of Yellow fever is involved in great obscurity, and many of the very highest European authorities believe that this disease was imported originally into the old world, and that it still may be transported from one country to another. There is no time here for discussing this point, and I will only say that the mass of authority in favor of this opinion is such as to challenge our full respect; no reasonable man, in the present state of facts, can assert positively that Yellow Fever may not under peculiar circumstances be transported.

I have shown that Yellow Fever often commences in a point from which it gradually extends from house to house for several weeks—now, it is clear, that in this case there must be a local, though invisible cause—it cannot exist in the atmosphere, as it could not, if thus diffused, be confined to a point. Suppose the infected point and a few surrounding acres of ground were taken up in August and put down in the centre of New-York or Philadelphia, is it not probable that the disease would spread from this point as in Mobile? If so, why may not the morbific cause be carried and thrown out of a vessel with a cargo of damaged coffee, potatoes, grain, sugar, meat, etc.? The germ might here find a hiding place, though I have no idea that the gaseous emanations from these vegetable or animal substances could produce Yellow Fever. We have no reason to believe that such emanations, differing so widely in themselves, can produce *one specific* disease.

We have evidence around us almost constantly that the germs of Insects lie dormant for indefinite periods and are then suddenly called into activity and propagated with inconceivable rapidity. By what physical causes these sleeping and waking states are governed, human sagacity cannot yet divine.

Involved in equal mystery are the habits, mode of propagation, etc., of contagious diseases. Small Pox, for example, is a highly *contagious* disease, and yet has its periods of activity and repose—at one time it disappears entirely—at another a few sporadic cases are seen—again we see it scattered irregularly here and there, and lastly it comes as a great Epidemic sweeping over a whole nation.

Small Pox, though known in China 2000 years earlier, was not carried to Europe until somewhere about the beginning of the 8th century A. D., and the fact is equally certain that it was not known in America until brought here by Columbus. There are strong reasons for believing that Scarlatina and Measles were also imported from Asia—yet these diseases have become perfectly domesticated in this country, and preserve all their ancient habits. Every now and then we hear of cases of Small Pox, occurring in localities removed from the thoroughfares, where it has never been known before, and under circumstances which render it impossible to trace its origin—still it must be carried to such points, for the disease is only propagated by *contagion*, as it was unknown in Europe or America till imported.

Small Pox, Scarlatina, Typhus, etc., are transported not only in their mature form, but in the form of fomites. In the latter case the germ is united in some way to clothes, furniture and other inanimate substances, for indefinite periods, probably for years, and then from unknown causes is roused into activity. Typhus is sometimes carried about and spread in its most malignant form by persons who are not affected by the disease—the memorable instance of the *Black assizes*, Old Bailey, in 1750, when the Lord Mayor, two of the judges and other eminent persons, took the disease from prisoners and died of it, is often alluded to.

"It is probable that Yellow fever is caused by an insect or animalcule bred on the ground, and in what manner it makes its impression on the system, is but surmise—unless the animalcule is, like that of Psora, bred in the system, we could no more expect it to be contagious, than the bite of a serpent. We may therefore easily understand, that it can at the same time be transportable in the form of a germ, and yet not contagious."

Without wishing to take so broad a ground as insect origin for all, I must say that those diseases arising from morbid poisons, present strong analogies with insect life. The Itch is a contagious disease which may be transported from place to place in all seasons and all climates, and is unquestionably *propagated by insects.* Like other contagious and epidemic diseases it prefers filthy places and persons of filthy habits. Other cutaneous affections have their origin in animalculæ, and M. Donné, one of the best microscopic observers of the day, asserts that the pus of Buboes contains animalcules, which account for the transmissibility of Syphilis.

Having no favorite hypothesis to sustain, and no other end in view but truth, it is proper to state that I have never myself witnessed any facts which would add much strength to the opinion that Yellow Fever is transmissible. There is, however, a mass of facts collected by numerous authorities on this point, which must be received at least with respect. The appearance and spread of this disease has often been mysteriously connected with the arrival of vessels from Yellow Fever ports—as in the case of the black assizes, a vessel might originate the disease, though no case had occurred on board during or before a voyage. At the time I am writing, Yellow Fever has appeared in Mobile and New Orleans *a month earlier than it has been known* for a number of years, and in the midst of heavy rains which had fallen every day for a month preceding the disease. Vessels have been, for some months, in consequence of the Mexican war, coming, in unprecedented numbers, from Vera Cruz and other ports where Yellow Fever was prevailing. Now although we cannot point to the chain of cause and effect, the circumstances in connection with the strange habits of diseases known to be transmissible, are sufficient to excite suspicion.

The remarkable manner in which Yellow Fever occurs in our northern cities, where it does not dwell, and where the natives cannot be acclimated against it, would seem to lend support to the idea of importation. I do not recollect any *Epidemic* of this disease in Boston since 1693. In Philadelphia it had not been seen for more that thirty years previous to the memorable 1793, when it began to assume an activity hitherto unknown at the north; and in the latter part of that century and beginning of the present, it occurred frequently, not only in the large but the small inland towns, as Catskill, Winchester, Middletown, and numerous other points in the Eastern and Middle States. Since 1823 the disease has not been known north of Charleston, I believe, and it is difficult to assign reasons why it should have appeared so often in rapid succession and then disappear for a long series of years. If it depended on animal and vegetable putrefaction, such could not, I think, be its course. It would seem more probable that the germ of the disease, which is exotic, when transported to an uncongenial climate, may exist for a few years, but finally becomes exhausted and perishes. Let any one desirous of honestly investigating this subject read the thirty years war between the New York and Philadelphia schools, and he will find much material for sober reflection and doubt on the transmissibility of Yellow Fever.

Yellow Fever came at the north in 1793, and ravaged the towns almost without interruption, for a series of years, and no one can tell why or whence it came, or for what reason it has not been seen in New York and Philadelphia for more than twenty years. Nor can we tell from whence came the Hessian Fly, that appeared first in 1776, on Long Island, nor why it departed after laying waste the wheat fields for a number of years. It was called the Hessian fly, but its true origin I believe is yet unknown. This fly travelled only about fifteen miles a year until it passed from our land.

Dr. Rush makes the remark, that no practitioner in the United States is likely to meet with Scarlet Fever oftener than once during his lifetime, so rare was this disease in his day, and yet no Epidemic affection is now more common than this in our country. I never saw or heard of it in South Carolina (my native State) until about fifteen years ago, nor do I believe it ever occurred in the interior of that State before. My old preceptor, who had been in practice forty years, then saw it for the first time; and now it has been become domesticated there, and sporadic cases (like Yellow Fever here) are seen every year.

Dr. Hulse, the distinguished surgeon of the Naval Hospital in Pensacola, informed me in 1841, that he had been in that town eighteen years, and had never seen there a case of Scarlet Fever. Rochoux (a well known authority) mentions the singular fact that Scarlet Fever is unknown in the Antilles, and that the natives of these Islands *must live in France eighteen months or two years before they can become so acclimated as to become susceptible to this disease!*

It is difficult to say where is the *home* of Yellow Fever, but even in the West Indies it has its periods of repose and activity; sometimes lying dormant for ten years, as was the case from 1828 to 1838 in some of the islands. If it is a disease originally of *one* country, which has been transported to others, its native place is probably that where it occurs with most regularity.

It has been observed of those great Epidemics which traverse the globe (as Cholera, Influenza, &c.) that germs are left behind, which, for several years, give rise to sporadic cases of identical character; and it would not surprise me at any time to see the Cholera again spring up in an epidemic form in New Orleans. There are several well authenticated instances where it has recurred at successive periods in the same vessel, showing that a germ is left. Like the seventeen year locust, it might take a Rip Van Winkle sleep, and again awake to its work of destruction.

Those gentlemen who contend for the absolute non-transmissibility of Yellow Fever would do well to weigh these and all the facts of similar import, before they rudely condemn others of equal honesty and ability, holding opposite opinions. The argument is utterly inconclusive, though a thousand instances be proven that vessels or steamboats with Yellow Fever on board have gone to distant ports, or ascended the Alabama and Mississippi Rivers without spreading the disease. Half a dozen well authenticated facts to the contrary are amply sufficient to overthrow it. Yellow Fever, like many other diseases, cannot be propagated in certain localities where the local circumstances are uncongenial to it. You cannot carry it to the interior towns on the Alabama River because some local condition is wanting; still it would seem that the germ of the disease lurks about steamboats, as in those seasons when Yellow Fever prevails in Mobile, it appears almost invariably in the old boats lying up and repairing on the Bay or Rivers within ten or fifteen miles of the town. Small Pox is known to be one of the most contagious of all diseases, and yet it has not extended in our city for the last twelve years, though vessels are bringing in cases every winter, and occasional sporadic cases are occurring which cannot be accounted for. How often too do we see solitary cases of Scarlet Fever occurring in families without contaminating other children, and we have already mentioned the fact that this disease cannot be propagated in the Antilles.

Can any one of the anti-contagionists explain why these contagious diseases are not communicable at one time, and so deadly at another? or why the Asiatic Cholera should suddenly assume an Epidemic form and encircle the globe?

In conclusion (on this point) I would remark, that admitting my suggestions to be true, they do not afford any ground for the vexatious and ruinous quarantine laws which have been enacted against Yellow Fever. A vessel *with Yellow Fever on board* should not be allowed to lie near a town, but here the restrictions should cease. If Yellow Fever is transportable by vessels at all, the instances are so rare, as not to justify very rigid quarantine regulations. Commerce is one of the *great necessities* of society, and law-makers should take into consideration the injuries as well as the benefits of their acts.

As, according to the theory we are discussing, the Natural History of Yellow Fever is closely allied to the Natural History of Insects, it is proper that I should say a few words more on the latter. The Infusoria, or Microscopic animalcules particularly demand a passing notice, as few of our readers have access to original sources on this curious subject. It has, I think, been pretty clearly shown that the propagation of

Yellow Fever cannot be explained by the Malarial theory, and it must remain with the reader to determine whether the chain of analogies offered, render the Insect theory more probable.

" Were a naturalist to announce to the world the discovery of an animal, which for the first five years of its life existed in the form of a serpent; which then, penetrating into the earth, and weaving a shroud of pure silk of the finest texture, contracted itself within this covering into a body without external mouth or limbs, and resembling more than any thing else an Egyptian mummy ; and which, lastly, after remaining in this state without food and motion for three years longer, should at the end of that period burst its silken cerements, struggle through its earthy covering, and start into day a winged bird—what think you would be the sensation excited by this strange piece of intelligence ?"—*Kirby and Spence—Entomology.*

Wonderful and incredible as this story would seem, it is but a faithful picture of what occurs in the *metamorphoses* of the Insect world. The beautiful butterfly that flits around us on a summer's day has passed through all these miraculous changes. First crawling from the egg, we see the *larva* (serpent)—next comes the *pupa* (mummy,) and lastly the butterfly, that might with much more propriety be ranked with the bird of Paradise than the disgusting catterpillar from which it sprung.

The microscopic wonders, revealed by Leeuwenhoek and other old writers, which for a long time were regarded, at best, only as honest delusions or creations of the imagination, have been thrown quite into the shade by modern discoveries ; but it is to the great work of Ehrenberg that we are more particularly indebted for our greatly augmented and more positive knowledge of *Infusoria.*

If a small portion of animal or vegetable matter (as a leaf or piece of flesh) be immersed in pure distilled water, and allowed to remain for a day or two, and a drop of the fluid be then placed under the focus of a powerful microscope, it is seen to swarm with myriads of animalcules which are termed *Infusoria.* A very faint idea may be conceived of the infinite extent of these minute forms of insect life from the simple fact stated by Ehrenberg, that five hundred millions (almost as many as the aggregate of the human race) may exist in a single drop of water !

The term *Infusoria* has been used as a generic one to embrace all microscopic *animalcula;* there are, however, forms which should not come under this head. Like the stars in the heavens, the number of their species increases just in proportion as our artificial vision is perfected, and we have every reason to believe that countless species still exist, too small to be reached by our most powerful microscopes. The infusoria proper, which are found in fluids, are of course more easily seized and examined than those minute microscopic beings that are floating through the air.

Ten years ago, Ehrenberg had described no less than 722 species of Infusoria, and many new ones have been added since that time. Already has observation gone so far as to make it seem possible that there is no form of matter which is not composed of living, dead, or fossil animalcula. Every breath of air we breathe, every particle of fluid or solid we swallow, all the water of the land and of the sea, every solid of the earth we tread upon, is known to abound with them. Many rocks, as the lime stone and cretaceous formations and whole geological strata are composed almost entirely of fossil animalcula ; even the solid gun flint is largely indebted to them. Ehrenberg has described 76 species of fossil Infusoria, belonging to 15 genera. It has even been asserted by a distinguished naturalist that the living muscles are composed of animalcules.*

When we stand before the fossil remains of the Mastodon or the monster Saurien of Alabama, we are lost in wonder at the magnitude and grandeur of the structure ; but far more wonderful and incompre- hensible in reality is the animalcule whose length is but the 30,000th part of an inch ! How is it possible, that a living animal, possessing all the complicated machinery necessary to animal life, can be crowded into a portion of space so infinitely small ? It has a head, with teeth—a body with an alimentary canal and complete digestive apparatus—a muscular system with the necessary organs of locomotion—organs of generation—in short, all the apparatus necessary for the existence of an independent being, relying upon external relations.

It is a common impression that Infusoria are found only in stagnant waters where putrefaction is going on, but this is a great mistake—it is true that they are more abundant in such situations, but they abound also in pure lakes, and in running streams, particularly around aquatic plants. The broad ocean too abounds with them, and its beautiful phosphores- cence, so often described, is attributable exclusively to myriads of these minute beings. Backer has described 8 species of these phosphores- cent animalcules.

We read of, red snow, the color of which is ascertained to arise from animalcules—also of water of various colors—the colors sometimes rising or falling, as the animalcules rise up or sink down. The filthy scum on stagnant pools is but a mass of infusoria ; and we are told that extensive and fatal epidemics occur occasionally amongst fish which are attributable to infusoria. Kirkby and Spence tells us that the " showers of blood" recorded by historians, are ascertained to be the excrement of a species of butterfly—one of the *Lepidoptera*—these showers cover every everything.

Though infusoria are most abundant in warm weather, they are also found in winter, beneath the ice, in frozen streams. The researches of Ehrenberg agree with those of Spalanzani, in showing that cold is dan- gerous generally to infusoria and especially to the *Rotatoria* (which are of the most perfect organization) and is more injurious to the living animal than their eggs—both the animal and the eggs perish by sudden heat, but sustain it better when gradually applied—some species support greater heat than others. These facts are interesting in connexion with certain experiments showing the disinfecting action of heat—contagious and epidemic diseases have been expelled and are best expelled from vessels, by closing them up and heating the confined air to a high tem- perature—*the germ of the disease is thus destroyed.*

* The various facts given are mostly on the authority of Ehrenberg, Mandl, Dujardin, Donne and Edwards—well known authorities.

Light is favorable to the production of Infusoria, but not indispensable, as some species are found in the deepest mines. *Too strong a light* is unfavorable to them and if our theory of Yellow Fever be correct, this may be the reason why the morbific cause is most active at night.

Infusoria are variously acted on by poisonous substances soluble in water—those of fresh water are instantly killed by a drop of salt water though the latter has myriads of its own. Strychnine and many other substances kill them instantly—they swallow Rhubarb with impunity—calomel, corrosive sublimate and camphor do not kill them for some hours. Wine and rum, as well as sugar, says M. Dujardin, kills a great many of those animalcules found in potable water,—a fact, with regard to which, the great mass of the population of Mobile would seem to have as strong an *instinct*, as had Jack Falstaff of the Blood Royal, if we are to judge by the immense amount of ingeniously contrived alcoholic compounds swallowed daily in our pious city.

Infusoria are bred in different ways—some are oviparous—some ovoviviparous—others viviparous ; lastly, many are gemmiparous and they propagate with inconceivable rapidity. Direct experiment has shown that we may obtain from a single one of the *Rotifers* (Rotatoria,) a million on the 10th; four millions on the 11th ; and sixteen millions on the 16th day ; and the progression is still more rapid in the Polygastric Infusoria. But perhaps the most prolific of all living things are some species of Aphides (plant-louse.) The following curious extract is from Kirkby and Spence's Entomology :—" As almost every animal has its peculiar *louse*, so has almost every plant its peculiar *plant-louse ;* and, next to locusts, these are the greatest enemies of the vegetable world, and like them are sometimes *so numerous as to darken the air.* The multiplication of these little creatures is infinite and almost incredible. Providence has endued them with privileges promoting fecundity, which no other insects possess ; at one time of the year they are viviparous, at another oviparous ; and what is most remarkable, and without parallel, the sexual intercourse of one original pair serves for all the generations which proceed from the female for a whole succeeding year. Reaumur has proved that in five generations one Aphis may be the progenitor of 5,904,900,000 (billions) descendants ; and it is supposed that in one year there may be 20 generations ! ! !"

With these few facts before us, how much more easily may we account for the spread of yellow fever from a focus, by the insect, than by the Malarial hypothesis—here is something tangible and comprehensible.

Not only the living, but *dead* animalcules *may* be a cause of disease—those who prefer this doctrine may, if they like, appropriate them in a putrifying mass to the support of their malarial notions.

In the May No. 1845, of the London Quarterly Journal of the Geological Society, may be found an exceedingly interesting article (taken from one by Ehrenberg in a Berlin Journal) " on the muddy deposits of the mouths of various Rivers, and the infusoria found in those deposits."

Ehrenberg has discovered in the mud now depositing " forms of Microscopic life and Infusoria identical even in species with those found in the fossil state in the oolitic and cretaceous ormations in every quarter of the globe."

It has already been stated that the fresh water and marine animalcules are entirely different, and Professor Ehrenberg has established the novel fact, that " the microscopic animalcules found in the marsh lands at the head of tide water in the Elbe (and so with other rivers) are the same as those in the ocean—possessing silicious and calcareous skeletons. These organic forms, which are better preserved at the depth of several feet, than on the surface, existed in the arable land of the valley of the Elbe, which had been accumulating for thousands of years, and in this way is explained the origin of this soil in a more satisfactory manner than has hitherto been attempted." The marine animalcules have been carried up with the tide, killed by the fresh water, and largely assisted in forming a deposit which heretofore has been attributed to the *river* deposit alone. The examination of the river at Gluckstadt and Hamburg has proved the existence there of 58 different species of marine animalcules.

Some idea may be formed of the extent of this putrifying mass, from the fact stated by Ehrenberg, that one cubic foot of every 20 of the alluvial islands of the Elbe is composed of animalcular remains, chiefly of marine origin. He states farther that the great bulk of the deposit is sand which under the microscope is found to be the *silicious shells* of extinct animalcules. From these facts it would seem that at least one half of the whole deposit is living, dead, and fossile animalcula. To these facts is attributable the fertility of these islands and marsh lands.

Yellow fever has a mysterious connexion with the seaboard and embouchures of rivers, but I will not pause to speculate on this point—it does occasionally wander a short distance from tide water and I have under the head of contagion explained the manner in which this might occur.

The habits and instincts of larger insects are obscured by numerous impediments, but how much more perplexing must be the natural history of those which can only be reached by powerful microscopes ? We have learned much about the infusoria proper, but myriads of minute beings might inhabit the air and even congregate in such numbers as to dim the light of the sun without our being able to seize and observe them. Denying animalcules the power of flight, which would be absurd, there are still ample provisions for their transportation long distances either in the form of egg or perfect animal. We have already seen how they are transported by water and by vessels, and there is reason to believe that they may be taken up with aqueous vapor and carried off by the winds. Even the Gossamer spider will sail upon his little web great distances. A shower of them fell upon the English vessel Beagle, in her voyage round the world a few years ago, when 60 miles from land,

To illustrate the influence which currents of wind may have in their distribution, the following facts are taken from an article in the Feb. No., 1845, of the London Quarterly Journal Geolog. Sciences, by the distinguished naturalist, Chas. Darwin, who made the voyage in the Beagle.

Many scattered accounts have appeared, concerning the dust which has fallen in considerable quantities on vessels at sea. great distances from land. Mr. Darwin has collected the details of 15 distinct instances in some of which dust fell for several days. It has several times fallen on vessels when between 300 and 600 miles from the coast of Africa; and it fell in May, 1840, on the Princess Louisa when 1030 miles from Cape Verd, the nearest point of the continent.

The instances related are given with such detail, and are so well authenticated as to leave no room as to their accuracy. The dust is often so abundant on the African coast as to cover every thing on board the vessels, as we often see dust over our furniture during spells of dry weather. Particles as large as the 1000th part of an inch have been blown to a considerable distance, on one occasion, 330 miles, and the atmosphere became hazy and the sun was dimmed. Mr. Darwin follows these facts by this remark—" The fact of particles of this size having been brought at least 330 miles from the land, is interesting as bearing on the distribution of the sporules of Cryptogamous plants and the ovules of Infusoria." Again he says, " Professor Ehrenberg has examined the dust collected by Lieut. James and myself, and he finds that it is, *in considerable part, composed of Infusoria, including no less than 67 different forms;* the little packet of dust collected by myself would not have filled a quarter of a tea-spoon, and yet it contained 17 forms.

One of the most highly organized and the most interesting in connection with our subject, is the *Rotifer*, (Rotatoria,) which is found not only in moist, but in perfectly dry places. It possesses the remarkable quality, first observed by Leeuwenhoek some 150 years ago, of remaining in a dry and apparently lifeless state for an indefinite period, and then being again resuscitated by the application of moisture. It is found not only in the parched sands of the plain, but in the dust of the gutters on the house tops, exposed to the burning summer sun. The application of moisture restores them immediately to life and activity.

Here we have the proof that both the animalcule and its germ may lie dormant, as is the habit of certain diseases, and then be brought into activity when its appropriate stimulus is applied. We have the evidence, too, that they may be transported through the air to a distant point, and there abide their time, as do the fomites which transport contagious diseases. What are the causes, meteorological or other, which call them into action, we are as ignorant as we are of those which govern larger insects, as the Aphides, the Hessian Fly, the Cotton Worms, &c., or as we are of the causes which regulate the temperature, the quantity of rain, or the electric states of the atmosphere, in different years.

It is difficult to conceive that the various forms of fever described should arise from a common source, and as chemistry has failed to detect a gas or emanation which can produce any one of them, their causes perhaps may be sought with more success in the different forms of Insect life. Works on Poisons have classified and thrown into separate groups those substances which have general resemblances in their modes of action; and so closely do articles of the same group similate each other in effects, that we are often much perplexed in distinguishing them. The Narcotic poisons, for example, though derived from different plants, and differing in their analysis, will often produce symptoms so alike as to render it impossible for us to decide, under which a patient is laboring. The same confusion will be found in the poisonous effects of different snakes, spiders, &c. In like manner, fevers, if arising from insects of the same *genus*, might present some general characteristics in common, and yet preserve *Specific* differences.

Ehrenberg, Mandl and Dujardin inform us that different animalcules are found in different localities. Stagnant waters on calcareous soils contain Infusoria which may be sought in vain in those of Argillaceous soils. The latter, ferruginous waters, those of turf, those of *ditches around habitations*, all have their peculiar inhabitants. Again, we may seek in vain for Infusoria in one season which are found in another, and no reason can be assigned for their appearance or disappearance. Here we have another analogy with the different types and habits of fevers.

The observations of Ehrenberg did not detect Infusoria in the dews, and yet there are strong reasons for believing that they exist here. By operating on moisture condensed from the atmosphere, Moschati, Guntz, Brocchi and Rigaud de Lisle, Vauquelin, Rigaud and Julia have shown incontestibly the presence of animal matter in air, and it is highly probable that it exists in an organic form. Some very well conducted experiments to the same effect have been made by Professor Riddell of New Orleans, which may be found in the Medical Journal of that city.

Professor Jackson, of Philadelphia, in a paper published by him in 1824, (I think, but it is mislaid,) informs us that during the last Epidemic of Yellow Fever in that city, the microscope detected immense numbers of animalcules in the Black Vomit, and none in the fluids ejected from the stomachs of those laboring under other fevers in the hospital at the same time.

We know that certain cutaneous diseases are produced by animalcules—that animalcules and little worms are very often found in the various fluids of the body, as the blood, urine, bile, &c.—also in the solids, as the brain, liver, eye, &c. Linnæus gives us a case of Dysentery, clearly produced by what he calls the *Acarus Dysenterica*. M. Donné, as before stated, has discovered in the pus of Buboes, animalcules which are constantly present, and which he regards as the cause of the transmissibility of Syphilis; and it is highly probable that the same discovery will yet be made for Small Pox, Plague, Cholera and other diseases. It is possible that Mercury and Iodine in Syphilis act as specifics, like sulphur does on Itch, by poisoning the animal cubs; and there is no reason why specifics might not be discovered for Yellow Fever and other diseases.

To one living on the Gulf of Mexico, it would look like a waste of time to speak of swarms and migrations of Insects. At the very moment I am writing I am annoyed by gnats, bugs, moths, &c., in such numbers that an inhabitant of a northern latitude could not conceive how I can connect two sentences together, and I confess that sometimes they are so troublesome that I am thinking more of my persecutors than the subject before me. Facts however that are before us constantly, cease to excite reflection, and it may be well to give a few prominent examples touching the *Migrations* of *Insects*.

At the moment I am writing I see by the newspapers that a brown fly of peculiar character, and which no one recollects to have seen before, has appeared in and around Cincinnati in immense clouds, covering the country for miles. No conjecture can be formed respecting their point of departure. Kirby and Spence give us the following account of gnats :

"We are told that in the year 1736, they were so numerous, that vast columns of them were seen to rise in the air from Salisbury Cathedral, which at a distance resembled columns of smoke, and occasioned people to think that the Cathedral was on fire. A similar occurrence, in like manner giving rise to an alarm of the church being on fire, took place in July, 1812, at Sagan, in Silesia. In the following year, at Norwich, in May, at about six o'clock in the evening, the inhabitants of the city were alarmed by the appearance of smoke issuing from the upper window of the spire of the Cathedral, for which at the time no satisfactory account could be given, but which was most probably produced by the same cause. And in the year 1776, in the month of August, they appeared in such incredible numbers at Oxford as to resemble a black cloud, darkening the air, and almost totally intercepting the beams of the sun." Even in "Lapland their numbers are so prodigious as to be compared to a flight of snow when the flakes fall thickest or to the dust of the earth."

The instincts by which insects are at certain times impelled to *emigration*, even to great distances, are very strange and unaccountable. Sometimes flights of them are met far out at sea. "De Geer has given an account of the larvæ of certain gnats, (Tipulariæ,) which assemble in considerable numbers for this purpose, so as to form a band of a finger's breadth, and from one to two yards in length. And what is remarkable while on their march, which is very slow, they adhere to each other by a kind of glutinous secretion ; but when disturbed, they separate without difficulty. Kuhn mentions another of the same tribe, the larvæ of which live in society and emigrate in files like the caterpillar of the procession moth. First goes one, then follow two, then three, &c., so as to exhibit a serpentine appearance, probably from their simultaneous undulating motion and the continuity of the files ; whence the common people in Germany call them *heerwurm*, and view them with great dread, regarding them as ominous of war. But of the Insect emigrants, none are more celebrated than the locusts, which, when arrived at their perfect state, assemble, as before related, in such numbers, as in their flight to intercept the sunbeams and to darken whole countries ; passing from one region to another, and laying waste kingdom after kingdom," &c.

But it is needless to multiply instances of this kind, and if any one should be at all incredulous, let him spend a night in a southern swamp. I will add one very singular example of the instinct of insects :

"There are annually two generations of the Angoumois Moth, an insect destructive to wheat. They first appear in May and June, and lay their eggs upon the ears of wheat in the fields ; the second appear at the end of summer in autumn and lay their eggs upon wheat in the granaries. These last pass the winter in the state of larvæ from which proceeds the first generation of moths. But what is extremely singular as a variation of instinct, those moths which are disclosed in May and June in the granaries, quit them with a rapid flight at sunset and betake themselves to the yet unreaped fields, where they lay their eggs; while the moths which are disclosed in the granaries after harvest, stay there and never attempt to go out, but lay their eggs upon the stored wheat. This is as extraordinary and inexplicable as if a litter of rabits produced in the spring were impelled by instinct to eat vegetables, while another produced in autumn should be as irresistibly directed to choose flesh."

The history of those great epidemics which sweep over the surface of the globe affords very strong support to the Insect theory. The Cholera, though not more remarkable than many other, may be selected for illustration. This disease, which started in Bengal, after assuming the epidemic form, travelled on until it arrived at the foot of the gigantic range of mountains which separates Asia from Europe—it seemed for several years unable to cross this immense barrier, but finally, like a river which had been pent up, it burst over into Russia in the dead of winter, when the mercury was almost freezing in the thermometer (and no doubt *quite* on the ridge of the mountains) and ravaged Moscow like a plague; and after 17 years of unceasing travel it completed the circle of the globe. Its general course may be followed from first to last, though there are many irregularities in the details—sometimes it turned to the right, sometimes to the left—now leaping over several hundred miles and passing on, or after a time retracing its steps and attacking towns which had congratulated themselves on an escape—usually preferring to follow great water courses and to prevail in summer, but at other times travelling over hills and sandy plains, and in the coldest weather. Wherever it prevailed, too, a tendency to reproduction remained for several years, as if germs were scattered in its track.

By what other than the Insect theory can these facts be explained?—No gas—no emanation—no form, in short, of inorganic matter could thus extend itself for 17 years around the globe, propagating as it travelled and scattering the seeds of reproduction behind it. All the theories which have been started, are absurd.

Sir Henry Holland, in tracing the erratic habits of insects in connection with this disease, says of them: "such are their frequent, sudden generation, at irregular and often distant periods, under certain circumstances of season and locality, or under other conditions less obvious to apprehension. The diffusion of swarms so generated and with rapidly repeated propagation over wide tracts of country and often following particular lines of movement," etc.

"Whatever is true as to the habits of insects obvious to our senses, is likely to be more especially so in those whose minuteness removes them farther from observation. Their generation may be presumed to be more dependent on casualties of season and place; their movements determined by causes of which we have less cognizance; and their power of affecting the human body to be in some ratio to their multitude and minuteness."—"Their direction to certain plants only—their settlements upon these in clusters and detached localities—the frequent suddenness of their change of place and disappearance, are all circumstances of curious analogy; as also the curiously abrupt limitation of some of those swarms, showing itself in definite lines of direction, along which their work of destruction is carried on."

Miasmatic fevers abound most in Southern latitudes and in marsh lands ; and the reason assigned is the greater amount of vegetable matter which is here subjected to rapid decomposition. But it should not be forgotten that here, too, are to be found in great excess the various forms of Insect life, Infusoria, etc., etc. Every plant not only has one parasite, but it is estimated that there is an average of six to each plant. Some idea may be formed of the immense number of insects in warm climates when it is stated that naturalists have variously estimated the number of species in the world at from 300,000 to 600,000.

Köllar tells us "that the distribution of Insects is in exact proportion to the diffusion of plants ; the richer any country is in plants, the richer it is also in insects. The polar regions which produce but few plants, have but few species of insects ; whereas the luxuriant vegetation of the tropical countries feeds a numerous host."

But it is high time that this long and rambling essay should be brought to a close. No one is more fully sensible of its imperfections than myself, but were I competent to do ample justice to the numerous topics alluded to, far more extended limits would be required than can here be permitted. The reader need not be told how endless and complicated are the ramifications of the subject of Malaria. I have not attempted to elaborate fully a single point, and my object has been simply to attract attention to certain phenomena of yellow fever which I think have been too much overlooked, and to lay before the profession, in connexion with them, some material which may serve for reflexion.

PUBLIC HEALTH
IN
AMERICA

An Arno Press Collection

Ackerknecht, Erwin H[einz]. **Malaria In the Upper Mississippi Valley: 1760-1900.** 1945

Bowditch, Henry I[ngersoll]. **Consumption In New England Or, Locality One of Its Chief Causes** and **Is Consumption Contagious, Or Communicated By One Person to Another In Any Manner?** 1862/1864. Two Vols. in One.

Buck, Albert H[enry] (Editor). **A Treatise On Hygiene and Public Health.** 1879. Two Vols.

Boston Medical Commission. **The Sanitary Condition of Boston:** The Report of a Medical Commission. 1875

Budd, William. **Typhoid Fever:** Its Nature, Mode of Spreading, and Prevention. 1931

Chapin, Charles V[alue]. **A Report On State Public Health Work,** Based On a Survey of State Boards of Health: Made Under the Direction of the Council on Health and Public Instruction of the American Medical Association. [1915]

Davis, Michael M[arks], Jr. and Andrew R[obert] Warner. **Dispensaries:** Their Management and Development. 1918

Dublin, Louis I[srael] and Alfred J. Lotka. **The Money Value of a Man.** 1930

Dunglison, Robley. **Human Health.** 1844

Emerson, Haven. **Local Health Units for the Nation.** 1945

Emerson, Haven. **A Monograph On the Epidemic of Poliomyelitis (Infantile Paralysis) In New York City In 1916.** 1917

Fish, Hamilton. **Report of the Select Committee of the Senate of the United States On the Sickness and Mortality On Board Emigrant Ships.** 1854

Frost, Wade Hampton. **The Papers of Wade Hampton Frost, M.D.:** A Contribution to Epidemiological Method. 1941

Gardner, Mary Sewall. **Public Health Nursing.** 1916

Greenwood, Major. **Epidemics and Crowd Diseases:** An Introduction to the Study of Epidemiology. 1935

Greenwood, Major. **Medical Statistics From Graunt to Farr.** 1948

Hartley, Robert M. **An Historical, Scientific and Practical Essay On Milk, As an Article of Human Sustenance:** With a Consideration of the Effects Consequent Upon the Unnatural Methods of Producing It for the Supply of Large Cities. 1842

Hill, Hibbert Winslow. **The New Public Health.** 1916

Knopf, S. Adolphus. **Tuberculosis As a Disease of the Masses & How To Combat It.** 1908

MacNutt, J[oseph] Scott. **A Manual for Health Officers.** 1915

Richards, Ellen H. [Swallow]. **Euthenics:** The Science of Controllable Environment. 1910

Richardson, Joseph G[ibbons]. **Long Life and How To Reach It.** 1886

Rumsey, Henry Wyldbore. **Essays On State Medicine.** 1856

Shryock, Richard Harrison. **National Tuberculosis Association 1904-1954:** A Study of the Voluntary Health Movement In the United States. 1957

Simon, John. **Filth-Diseases and Their Prevention.** 1876

Sternberg, George M[iller]. **Sanitary Lessons of the War and Other Papers.** 1912

Straus, Lina Gutherz. **Disease In Milk:** The Remedy Pasteurization. The Life Work of Nathan Straus. 1917

Wanklyn, J[ames] Alfred and Ernest Theophron Chapman. **Water Analysis:** A Practical Treatise on the Examination of Potable Water. 1884

Whipple, George C. **State Sanitation:** A Review of the Work of the Massachusetts State Board of Health. 1917. Two Vols. in One.

Selections From Public Health Reports and Papers Presented at the Meetings of the American Public Health Association (1873-1883). 1977

Selections From Public Health Reports and Papers Presented at the Meetings of the American Public Health Association (1884-1907). 1977

Animalcular and Cryptogamic Theories On the Origins of Fevers. 1977

The Carrier State. 1977

Clean Water and the Health of the Cities. 1977

The First American Medical Association Reports On Public Hygiene In American Cities. 1977

Selections from the Health-Education Series. 1977

Health In the Southern United States. 1977

Health In the Twentieth Century. 1977

The Health of Women and Children. 1977

Minutes and Proceedings from the First, Second, Third and Fourth National Quarantine and Sanitary Conventions. 1977. Four Vols. in Two.

Selections from the Journal of the Massachusetts Association of Boards of Health (1891-1904). 1977

Sewering the Cities. 1977

Smallpox In Colonial America. 1977

Yellow Fever Studies. 1977